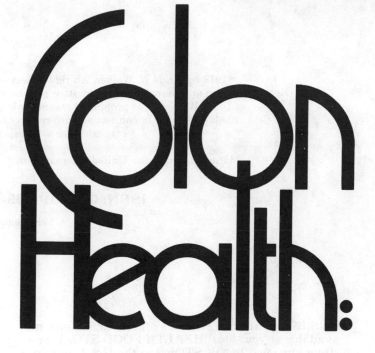

the KEY
to a
VIBRANT
LIFE

**Norman W. Walker,
D.Sc., Ph.D.**

ISBN: 0-89019-069-0

15th Printing

THIS BOOK, and Dr. Walker's other publications, are
available at your local HEALTH FOOD STORE and
from any good BOOK STORE in the U.S.A. and in
many countries abroad.

Should you have difficulty obtaining any book, you may
send your order direct to:

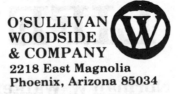

O'SULLIVAN
WOODSIDE
& COMPANY
2218 East Magnolia
Phoenix, Arizona 85034

ii

You don't need to relate your health to your age! For over seventy years Norman W. Walker, Ph.D., has proven through research that well-being and long life can go hand-in-hand. Modern day nutritionists and medical researchers are just now discovering the truths which Dr. Walker has known and expounded throughout the twentieth century. Dr. Walker himself is living proof that a longer, healthier life may be achieved through proper diet, mental soundness, and intelligent body care. Every year we read about a new fad diet, a "cure-all" drug, a food supplement, or a revolutionary exercise program that will save our lives. The Dr. Walker program is unique in that it doesn't use the promotional words, "miracle, fad, or revolutionary," ..... it doesn't need them!

Dr. Walker's contributions to our living longer, healthier lives began around the turn of the century in London, where as a young man he became seriously ill from over-work. Unable to accept the idea of ill health or a sick body, Dr. Walker cured himself. Since that time, he has successfully spent the last 70 years researching man's ability to extend life and achieve freedom from disease.

In 1910, Dr. Walker established the Norwalk Laboratory of Nutritional Chemistry and Scientific Research in New York, and thus began his important contributions to a longer, more active form of living. Among his great contributions was the discovery of the theraputic value of fresh vegetable juices, and in 1930 the development of the Triturator Juicer.

Today, Dr. Walker spends his entire work day continuing his research and writings. His book sales have reached the three million mark, and two new books are almost completed.

We believe Dr. Walker is the world's leading nutritionist; his unique contributions are all available to you through his books.

Colon Health:

YOU CAN REGAIN
the VITALITY
of YOUR YOUTH.

Contents

Contents

"I can truthfully say that I am never conscious
of my age. Since I reached maturity I have never
been aware of being any older, and I can say,
without equivocation or mental reservation, that
I feel more alive, alert, and full of enthusiasm
today than I did when I was 30 years old. I
still feel that my best years are ahead of me. I
never think of birthdays, nor do I celebrate them.
Today I can truthfully say that I am enjoying
vibrant health, I don't mind telling people how
old I am: I AM AGELESS!"

Norman W. Walker, D.SC., Ph.D.
Page 9; Vibrant Health

Illustrations

The Story Of The Solon Concerning His Colon

When he was a lad he had pains in his tummy,
　He had cramps so bad that he called for his Mummy.
She put him to bed, made him drink caster oil.
　From that day to this from that oil he'll recoil.

When late in his teens pimples covered his face.
　Something was wrong. He was a disgrace!
Surreptitiously he went to see a physician
　Who told him his sewage did not get recognition.

"I don't understand," he said, "I feel fine within."
　He was told, "Your sewage is coming out of your skin.
If you don't watch your food, keep your bowel free,
　You may be a dead duck in two years or three."

Then he said, "Don't ever eat or drink trash.
　Eat raw foods and drink juices, and save up your cash.
Take colonics regularly, as long as you live,
　About twice a year. That's the advice that I give."

He followed the old physician's advice.
　That has saved him many a bad habit and vice.
Today he is YOUNG — at 75,
　Full of energy and vigor. It's great to be alive!

N. W. Walker

Chapter 1.
The Colon And The Health Of Your Body

Your Body Needs Attention

Your body is the house in which you live. By analogy, it is just like the building in which you make your home. Your home needs, at the very least, periodical attention, otherwise the roof may leak, the plumbing may get out of order and clog up, termites will drill through the floors and the walls, and other innumerable cases of deterioration will make their appearance. Such is the case with your physical body. Every function and activity of your system, day and night, physical, mental, and spiritual, is dependent on the attention you give to it.

The kind and the quality of the food you put into your body is of vital importance to every phase of your existence. Good nutrition not only regenerates and rebuilds the cells and tissues which constitute your physical body, but also is involved in the processes by which the waste matter, the undigested food, is eliminated from your body to prevent corruption in the form of fermentation and putrefaction. This corruption, if retained and allowed to accumulate in the body, prevents any possibility of attaining any degree of vibrant health.

HEAD, CHEST & ABDOMEN

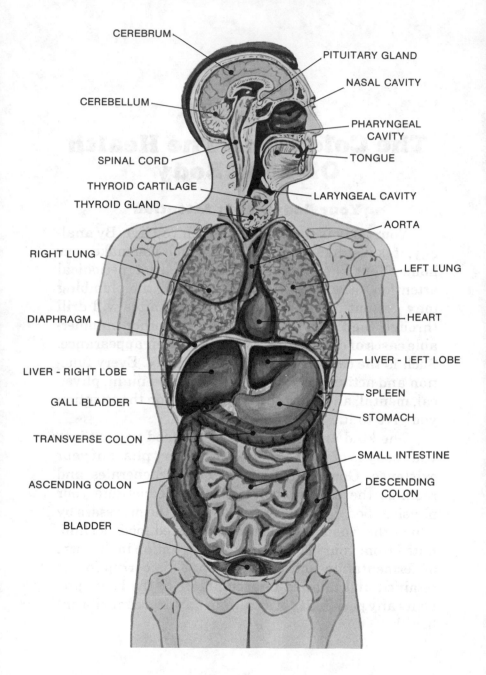

CEREBRUM

PITUITARY GLAND

NASAL CAVITY

CEREBELLUM

PHARYNGEAL CAVITY

TONGUE

SPINAL CORD

THYROID CARTILAGE

LARYNGEAL CAVITY

THYROID GLAND

AORTA

RIGHT LUNG

LEFT LUNG

DIAPHRAGM

HEART

LIVER - LEFT LOBE

LIVER - RIGHT LOBE

SPLEEN

GALL BLADDER

STOMACH

TRANSVERSE COLON

SMALL INTESTINE

ASCENDING COLON

DESCENDING COLON

BLADDER

The elimination of undigested food and other waste products is equally as important as the proper digestion and assimilation of food. In fact, because of the danger of the inevitable effects of toxemia, of toxic poisons, as the outcome of the neglected accumulation and failure to expel feces, debris, and other waste matter from the body, I can think of nothing more significant and vital! Few of us realize that failure to effectively eliminate waste products from the body causes so much fermentation and putrefaction in the large intestine, or **colon**, that the neglected accumulation of such waste can, and frequently does, result in a lingering demise!

Cause of Death? — Colon Neglect

The reality and importance of this colon problem was brought to my consciousness when I was a very young man. I was visiting an Aunt in Scotland when one morning a sudden piercing shriek ran through the house from the living room. There, on the floor, curled up in a paroxysm of agony, was my favorite cousin in her teens. The doctor, who was immediately called, declared she must have burst her appendix. She was rushed to the hospital in the family carriage in the company of the doctor, but she died within a few hours. The old doctor said he did not know what caused the appendix to burst; he was not taught in medical school that it is the natural result of neglecting the colon.* From that day to this, the colon has been the focal point of my research.

* The appendix, its care and relationship to the colon, will be discussed in a later chapter.

5

Your Colon and the Food You Eat

If a person has eaten processed, fried and over-cooked foods, devitalized starches, sugar and excessive amounts of salt, his colon cannot possibly be efficient, even if he should have a bowel movement two to three times a day! Instead of furnishing nourishment to the nerves, muscles, cells and tissues of the walls of the colon, such foods can actually cause starvation of the colon. A starved colon may let a lot of fecal matter pass through it, but it is unable to carry on the last of the digestive and nourishing processes and functions intended for it.

In order to live, the human body must be nourished. The cells and tissues composing the anatomy are live organisms with an amazing degree of resilience, elasticity and buoyancy. To be able to replenish and re-invigorate these cells and tissues, their nourishment must necessarily be composed of live elements, i.e., foods with life-giving properties. There are also foods whose ultimate function is to cleanse and remove used-up cells and tissues and pilot this waste matter to the colon for evacuation.

The bulk which is so essential for the proper and complete digestion of our food is needed in the colon just as much as in the small intestine. Such bulk, however, must be composed of fibers or roughage of raw foods. When these fibers pass through the intestines they become, figuratively speaking, highly magnetized, and in this condition are very helpful in the functions involved in the various parts of the intestines. In addition to receiving the residue of that part of our food which is not digested, the colon also accommodates itself to the fiber — the roughage — in the food upon which it depends for its "intestinal broom."

When the mineral elements which compose the foods we eat are saturated with oil or grease, the digestive organs cannot process them efficiently and they are passed out of the small intestine into the colon as debris. In addition, the body has a great deal of waste to dispose of through the colon in the form of used-up cells and tissues. When "demagnetized" food passes through the body system with little or no benefit, eventually, experience has proved, these foods leave a coating of slime on the inner walls of the colon like plaster on a wall. In the course of time this coating may gradually increase its thickness until there is only a small hole through the center, and the matter so evacuated may contain much undigested food from which the body derives little or no benefit. The consequent result is a starvation of which we are not conscious but which causes old age and senility to race towards us with the throttle wide open.

Civilization is built on the principle of financial gain. There is nothing wrong with financial gain, but when it is obtained at the expense of degenerating, vitiating and polluting our food, then we have no one to blame if we suffer the consequences of eating such food. Infirmity and sickness, at any age, is the direct result of loading up the body with food which contains no vitality, and at the same time allowing the intestines to remain loaded with waste matter.

The Colon — your Body's Sewer

The colon is a natural breeding ground for bacteria. The purpose and function of this bacteria is to neutralize, dissipate, avoid and prevent a toxic condition from developing in the colon. However, there are two types of bacteria: namely, the healthy, scavenging type known as bacilli coli, and the pathogenic or disease-producing kind. In a proper, clean, healthy environment the healthy scavenging bacteria will control the pathogenic kind. When too much fermentation and putrefaction is generated in the colon due to neglecting to keep it as free from feces and waste as possible, the pathogenic bacteria proliferate and ailments result. Such waste must necessarily be expelled from the body, and for this purpose your colon is equipped with a very efficient eliminative system. That is to say, "efficient" if it is in good and proper working order, functioning on the schedule suited to your physical condition.

The very best of diets can be no better than the very worst if the sewage system of the colon is clogged with a collection of waste and corruption. It is impossible, when we eat two, three, or more meals in a day, not to have residue accumulating in the colon in the form of undigested food particles, as well as the endproduct from food which has undergone digestion. Furthermore, not only does food-waste accumulate in the colon, but also the millions of cells and tissues which have served their purpose and have been replaced. These cells and tissues are dead proteins of a highly toxic nature if allowed to ferment and putrefy. You no

8

doubt have experienced the offensive aroma emanating from the body of an animal which has died and whose carcass has begun to decompose. The cells and tissues in the anatomy undergo the same decomposition when they are allowed to remain in the colon longer than necessary.

The very purpose of the colon as an organ of elimination is to collect all fermentative and putrefactive toxic waste from every part of the anatomy and, by the peristaltic waves of the muscles of the colon, remove all solid and semi-solid waste from the body.

In simple words, the colon is the sewage system of the body. Nature's laws of preservation and hygiene require and insist that this sewage system be cleansed regularly, under penalty of the innumerable ailments, sicknesses and diseases that follow, as the night follows the day, if waste is allowed to accumulate. Not to cleanse the colon is like having the entire garbage collecting staff in your city go on strike for days on end! The accumulation of garbage in the streets creates putrid, odoriferous, unhealthy gases which are dispersed into the atmosphere.

NORMAL COLON
SPHINCTERS and SACCULATIONS
and their
INTERRELATION
WITH ANATOMICAL CENTERS and PATHOLOGY

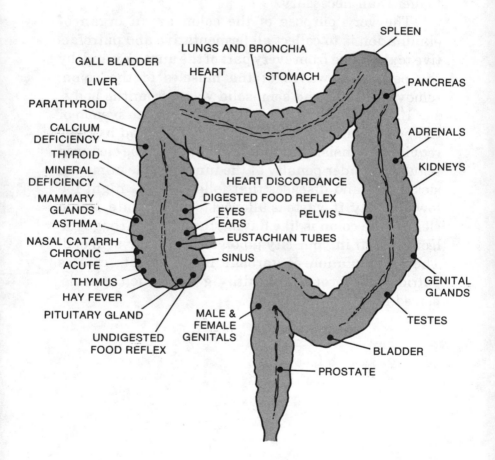

Chapter 2.
Constipation —
Your Body's Greatest Enemy

What Is Constipation?

The expression **constipation** is derived from the Latin word "constipatus," which translated means "to press or crowd together, to pack, to cram." Consequently, to be constipated means that the packed accumulation of feces in the bowel makes its evacuation difficult. However, a state of constipation can also exist when movements of the bowel **may seem to be normal**, in spite of an accumulation of feces somewhere along the line in the colon!

The fact of the matter is that constipation is the number one affliction underlying nearly every ailment; it can be imputed to be the initial, primary cause of nearly every disturbance of the human system. The most prevalent ailment afflicting civilized people is constipation. It is vital to stress that constipation affects the the health of the **colon**, upon which the health of the body in its entirety depends.

There are two crimes against Nature which civilization indulges in as a daily routine, which beget this, the most common and popular of our ailments, constipation. One is the consumption of devitalized and refined foods which fail to nourish the organs responsible for the evacuation of waste matter. The other, which is most prevalent particularly among young people, but not much less among the older and more mature, is neglecting to stop everything we are doing when the urge to evacuate the bowels should drive us headlong into the bathroom. Nature is a strict taskmaster; she gives one warning — sometimes two. You obey — or else. That "or else" is the insidious path to constipation.

How Constipation Effects the Colon's Function

If solving the problem of constipation were merely a case of washing out loose material lying free inside any part of the colon, it would not be too great a difficulty to clear the situation. A high enema would most likely be sufficient to take care of its removal. The problem, however, is not quite so simple to dispose of. Constipation involves not only the unnecessary retention of feces in the bowel, but also the retention present throughout the first half of the colon, from the cecum to the middle of the transverse colon. The cecum is found next to the ileo cecal valve at the beginning of the colon. (Please refer to the fold-out *Colon Therapy Chart* in the back of this book.)

The wall of this section of the colon is equipped with sensitive nerves and muscles whose function it is to create wavelike motions, known as peristaltic waves, to propel the contents of the colon from the cecum to the rectum for eventual evacuation. This is a distance of approximately five feet. If you will refer to the *Colon*

12

Therapy Chart you will see that the cecum is that part of the ascending colon at the exit of the small intestine, and the rectum is the lower bowel.

Besides the formation of these peristaltic waves, this first half of the colon has two other very important functions. First, it must extract from all the residue coming from the small intestine any available nutritional material which the small intestine was unable to collect. For this purpose, it mulches the material which passes into it from the small intestine and transfers the liquid and other elements through its walls into the blood stream. The nutrition which has thus been extracted from the colon is collected by the blood vessels lining the walls of the colon and is carried to the liver for processing.

Obviously, if the feces in the colon have putrefied and fermented, any nutritional elements present in it would pass into the blood stream as polluted products. What would otherwise be nutritional becomes, in fact, the generation of **toxemia**. Toxemia is a condition in which the blood contains poisonous products which are produced by the growth of pathogenic, or disease-producing, bacteria. Pimples, for example, are usually the first indication that toxemia has found its way into the body.

The other important function of the first half of the colon is to gather from the glands in its walls the intestinal flora needed to lubricate the colon. Far too many people, professional and laymen, think that enemas and colon irrigations wash out the intestinal flora and thus deprive the colon of a valuable means of lubrication. This school of thought is utterly false and totally devoid of truth and fact. Obviously, when the packed accumulation of feces in the bowel leads to fecal incrustation, it is not possible for the lining of the colon to function normally, and the glands in this lining cannot produce the necessary intestinal flora, or lubrication. Such lack of lubrication only serves to intensify a state of constipation and to generate toxemia.

This fecal incrustation interferes with, if it does not actually prevent, the infusion of the necessary intestinal flora for colon lubrication, the formation of peristaltic waves for evacuation purposes, and the absorption and use of the additional nutritional elements present in the waste residue coming into the colon from the small intestine.

It does not require much imagination to perceive that the adhesive quality of the feces in the colon is readily susceptible to creating a coating on the inside of the lining or wall of the colon, resembling a layer of plaster in its consistency. It is equally obvious that such a coating, in preventing the normal function of the colon, has the insidious effect of becoming a generator of toxicity, to the detriment of health, happiness and longevity.

A Hospital Stay. . . Canceled

Just a few years ago, a good friend of ours telephoned me from Indiana to tell me that he was scheduled to go into the hospital the next day. "What for?" I asked him. He told me he had a blocked colon and could not defecate. The prolonged retention of

14

feces and stale waste matter in the colon may, and frequently does, result in the blocking of the passage within the colon, making it impossible to have a bowel movement. I asked my friend why, knowing our program, he did not get some colon irrigations. "Oh," he answered, "that's out of the question. The nearest one is 100 miles from here." I told him I would travel 1,000 miles for some colonics before I would allow myself to be taken to the hospital!

As it turned out, my friend took that 100-mile trip and telephoned me a week or so later to say it had saved his life. He was feeling better than he had felt in years, and was going back for some more colonics soon. This is by no means an isolated case; I could fill a book with similar ones.

My study and intensive research on this subject convinces me more than ever that **no** treatment or healing procedure should **ever** be started without first giving the patient a series of colon irrigations in order to clean out the colon and remove the incipient source of infection. There is no ailment, sickness or disease that will not respond to treatment quicker and more effectively than it will after the administration of a series of colon irrigations.

Chapter 3.
Colon Therapy
Just Exactly What Is a Colon Irrigation?

After the plaster-like coating has definitely formed on the walls of the colon, not any number of high enemas will efficiently dissolve it. Furthermore, to remove it too rapidly would cause the inner lining of the colon to become "raw" and painful. Like the removal of plaster, the fecal coating in the colon must be thoroughly soaked and saturated with just plain water in order that its removal may take place gradually, comfortably, and effectively. This can be accomplished by a series of colon irrigations.

A colon irrigation is administered by an operator trained and accustomed to this work. You can look in the Yellow Pages of the telephone directory for listings under *Colonics* or *Colon Irrigations*. Also consult **Naturopaths**, **Chiropractors** and **Physiotherapists** and ask them if they have colonic equipment.

Colonics are, in effect, glorified enemas using many gallons of water — only a pint or two at a time — and are given by the colonic operator, usually a nurse, with the water flow and expulsion under the control of the operator, while the patient lies relaxed on an appropriate table which is connected with the colonic equipment. To be efficient, a colon irrigation requires a period of half an hour to one hour; during that period,

20 or 30 gallons of water may have been inserted into the colon through the rectum, at the rate of only one pint to perhaps two quarts of water at a time, then expelled each time. The first two or three irrigations can prove how sensible and comfortable the procedure actually is.

However, the best colonic equipment available can yield very poor and unsatisfactory results if the operator is inefficient because of a deficiency in the knowledge of the human anatomy. Therefore, the most important and vital adjunct to good colonic equipment is the employment of a knowledgeable, trained operator.

It is not enough to know all about colons and the principles of irrigation. The operator should also be familiar with the art of **foot relaxation**. Just as every part of the anatomy has nerve endings which are directly or indirectly associated with the colon, as I have indicated on the *Colon Therapy Chart*, so are the soles of the feet related, directly or indirectly, to every part of the anatomy, as I have indicated in the *Foot Relaxation Chart*. I strongly recommend that every colonic equipment installation should include these two charts, framed and hung on the wall facing the operator.

In examining this Foot Relaxation Chart you will notice that the center of the sole of each foot corresponds to the midriff and especially to the colon.

When the operator is functioning at the colonic table, he (or she) should massage the patient's feet — right and left sole in turn, with a fair amount of finger

17

pressure. In the beginning, as a general rule, this may result in the patient feeling a sharp pain. When this happens, it is an indication that uric acid crystals have accumulated in that spot on the foot, and the pressure causes the sharp points of these uric acid crystals to penetrate the nerves, resulting in a painful reaction. When such pain occurs, it is a definite indication that there is an excessive amount of fecal matter plastered on the inner wall of the colon. Gentler massage of these painful spots will react on the nerves of the colon and help the presence of the water in the colon to work more efficiently.

For some years there has been quite a campaign to try to induce colonic establishments to install equipment to inject oxygen into the colon together with the water. The immediate effect of this oxygen is invigorating, like a hypodermic needle shot in the arm would be. But I am more interested in the long-range results and effects. Almighty God gave man an excellent set of lungs by means of which the body could obtain the natural fresh air, which is composed of about 20% oxygen and about 80% nitrogen. It is a well-known clinical fact that there are certain kinds of lung troubles whereby the injection of oxygen into the **lower** part of the lungs is fatal. In a matter of 10 to 20 minutes the patient turns blue. Unless such an oxygen injection is immediately changed to the injection of air, the patient will die.

In my many score years of intimate study of the human anatomy I have never yet found any gland, organ or gadget which Nature has provided for oxygen to enter the colon, except what oxygen is already pres-

18

ent in the water entering the body through the rectum, and the natural moisture in the colon.

As a matter of fact, I have seen herons and other similiar birds in Florida stand by a river or pool of water, fill their long beaks, and inject water into the rectum in order to give themselves an enema or colon irrigation. I never asked these birds what school, college or university they went to in order to learn this principle of internal lavage.

Considering the long- range effect of injecting oxygen into the colon during an irrigation, I am not at all satisfied that there may not be some adverse effects eventually. A good sales talk is always convincing, particularly when one is not familiar with all the circumstances involved. Personally, I would never permit anyone to inject oxygen into my body, certainly not as a therapeutic answer to sales talks. I have had many scores, perhaps hundreds, of colon irrigations with nothing whatever added to the water and I intend to continue to do so.

When all is said and done, Almighty God furnished **air** and **water** as natural elements essential to human existence. For man's protection, **air** is composed of 20% oxygen and no more. More would have been excessive for our well-being. Just think — only one part oxygen plus four parts nitrogen! **Water** is composed of twice as much hydrogen as oxygen, also for man's protection; too much oxygen can kill. Common sense, if not clinical guess work, confirms the conclusion that unnecessary injections of oxygen have potential dangers. Of course there are conditions when, due to some deficiency or disturbance, we may need more oxygen than the lungs can supply, but in such a case oxygen is administered into the **lungs, not** into the rectum!

Of course, as you would expect, there are people who deplore the idea of internal cleansings. Some even have developed the mistaken notion that colon irrigations are beneficial only when accompanied by a long fast. This, as a matter of fact, is a fairly speedy way to undermine and devitalize the body. When the body is left without nourishment for more than six or seven days, the hungry cells and tissues become cannibalistic and feed on each other.

It is not for me to tell you what you must and what you must not do. Just use your God-given intelligence, and keep your internal organs clean and intact. After all, it's **your** body.

It is **very** important that a trained operator be constantly present during the administration of a colon irrigation. The patient should never be subjected to discomfort. One person may have an easy capacity for two quarts of water at one time, while another patient may not be able to tolerate more than one pint at a time because of the condition of the colon. For patients with a limited water capacity, it is also an advantage for the operator to have an X-ray picture of the patient's colon to consult while administering the colon irrigation. However, I do not recommend X rays unless they are absolutely necessary for the colon irrigation to be administered without undue discomfort to the patient.

Do not expect one or two colon irrigations to revitalize your system if you have neglected to take care of its excreta for 20, 30, or even 60 or 80 years, any more than you would expect a pill to cause all your ailments and troubles to vanish overnight.

Based on several score years of experience, research and observation, it is my considered opinion that every mature man and woman, irrespective of their degree of intelligence, should be quick to realize that if they have any desire to live a long and healthy life — and to prevent the decadence and degeneration of senility — they should seriously consider their condition and take a series of colon irrigations (by the dozens if necessary) and get started on this cleansing program. It took many years to accumulate whatever corruption that has adhered to the inside walls of your colon; therefore, give the irrigations the chance to cleanse you thoroughly. Thereafter, I am convinced that about twice a year, throughout life, colon irrigations should help Nature keep the body healthy. Bear in mind that colon irrigations are less expensive than hospitalization and surgeon's fees, and more certain of beneficial results!

And What About Diarrhea?

Diarrhea is the antithesis, or reverse, of constipation. It is a condition of frequent and fluid evacuations of the bowel. There are several types of diarrhea. Among these, the most usual is inflammatory diarrhea caused by the congestion of mucus in the colon, following the rapid chilling of the skin of the entire body, causing supression of perspiration, and in the case of a

21

female, slowing down menstruation. Another type of diarrhea is pancreatic, a persistent form, of a thin, ropy or glutenous consistency, due to a disturbance of the pancreas. There is also parasitic diarrhea, which is incited by the presence of intestinal parasites.

Every type of diarrhea I have had occasion to study has responded to colon irrigations when the patient submitted to them. This sounds like a contradiction in terms, but let me give you just one of several instances which have come under my direct notice.

There was a case of a woman who had been afflicted with very severe diarrhea for six or seven years, without any relief. She was also troubled with an inability to urinate. She submitted to drugs, medicines, and injections, but to no avail. She had been given enough shots to kill a rhinocerous, and every one of them made her more sick than ever.

She consulted a doctor friend of mine who asked me to give him my opinion. As soon as I saw her I told my friend that if I were in his place I would immediately start giving her colonic irrigations. Both he and his patient laughed at the very thought of such a procedure. However, we took an X-ray picture that confirmed my suspicion, and he finally agreed to try some colonics, although still declaring that a colonic was intended for a stoppage of the bowel and not for such a copious running-off. In less than 6 colonics she expelled some 15 pounds of stale fecal matter. Her diarrhea then gradually ceased, and the removal of the fecal impactions, which were crowding the colon against the bladder, enabled the passage of the urine to become normal.

I never lose an opportunity to emphasize the fact that unless we know definitely what the condition of our colon is, as indicated in the outline of two or more X-ray pictures, we cannot afford to deceive ourselves into thinking that it is all right. If we are eating foods that are cooked or processed, several bowel movements a day are *not* a sufficient indication that all is well.

The Dangerous Business of Laxatives and Cathartics

Laxatives and cathartics are "big business." This is evident in the prevalence of constipation. What happens when one takes such laxatives and cathartics? The result is usually the ejection of debris from the bowel. But why did this take place? Simply because the colon became so irritated in expelling the offending laxative that anything else that was loose went out with it. We have found that the use of laxatives and cathartics are not only habit forming but decidedly destructive to the membrane of the intestines. Laxatives and cathartics disturb the normal rhythm of the excretory organs, which sooner or later rebel. That is why so many people start with mild laxatives and soon graduate to cathartics before they reach the point of no return. This is where one gets a ticket for a colostomy!

The most striking result of a laxative addiction came to me in the person of a veteran. He was in his mid-thirties and came directly from the Veteran's Hospital in San Francisco to see me. Briefly, his history is this:

He had intended to make the Army his

23

career. Being afflicted with constipation, his doctor prescribed laxatives. These became progressively less effective until he was sick and down on his back. Specialists made many tests, finally deciding that by removing all his teeth it might cure him! It did not! Finally an exploratory operation brought to light the almost complete blockage of his colon. A colostomy followed, and he was given a permanent discharge from the Army. I gave him what advice I could and he left.

Back in San Francisco he improved somewhat, enough to look for employment. He had an appointment with one of the executives of a large corporation and promptly presented himself in the executive's plush, carpeted office. At the conclusion of the interview, as he was about to leave, the bottom of his colostomy bag opened, spilling its contents on the carpet! The young man rushed home to his sister, with whom he was living, and explained to her exactly what had happened. He then went into his room and put a bullet through his head. His sister gave me these tragic details.

Watch your colon!

Realize that a surgeon is trained to cut and amputate. It is not within his field to wash out the colon, or have it done. It is not surprising that nearly all (probably without exception) who have been afflicted with a colostomy never knew what was in store for them until

24

they awakened from the operation. Then, to their chagrin, they knew the full implications of a colostomy.

Be prudent. Be wise. Prevention is better than **no
cure**. Don't take my word for it. Prove it yourself by
taking a number of colonics. My own life will not be
affected in the least by what you do or don't do. But the
life it may save could be **yours**.

A Healthy Colon — A Lifetime Procedure

In the preceding pages we have learned how
vitally important it is to keep the colon clean and
washed out periodically. We will now study the mysterious and miraculous manner by which certain areas of
the colon are both directly and indirectly related to the
various organs and glands throughout the anatomy.
What could a pimple have to do with the colon? What
does eye, ear, or throat trouble have to do with the
colon? How can the colon possibly have anything to do
with the head, the feet, the heart or the glands? When
there is a disturbance in any particular area of the
colon, we can tell in which part of the anatomy an
affliction is present, or likely to appear. The colon is
intimately related to every cell and tissue in the body,
as you will learn by the time you finish studying this
book.

On the face of it, this statement seems absurd.
However, we must consider that our troubles started at
birth, soon after we inhaled our first breath. Did Mama
watch how and what the baby's bowel was evacu-
ating? Regularity of the bowel should start at birth and
continue until the autopsy indicates to what extent we

25

have cared for or neglected the attention the colon must have. Generally, progressive degeneration of the colon begins shortly after birth; a normal baby's colon is perfect, for a while. From childhood through adolesence, discipline (or the lack of it) is greatly responsible for its condition. Thereafter, knowledge and free-will determine the condition of the colon and its effect on the individual's physical, mental and spiritual health throughout the rest of his life.

I invite you to study every part of this book in the same state of consciousness that enables you to realize the miracle of your radio or television. Just think what mere man has accomplished in this day and generation! He has been able to condense and harness cosmic energy from the vast expanse of the universe into a tiny box we call our radio. With the radio we can channel the cosmic energy vibrations, or waves, by the mere turning of a little knob. Wherever you are, in your home or office, you can hear symphony music or listen to talks taking place 3,000, 6,000 or 10,000 miles away. Marvelous? If man can invent and discover such wonderful things, did not God Almighty do something that is infinitely greater when He formed man out of the dust of the earth with an electronic system that far surpasses anything man can do?

Just think, right here on my desk I have a little box with numbers and figures on "keys." I press the keys with certain numbers in rotation, then add, subtract, multiply, divide or do some other mathematical calculation, and the correct answer appears in a window in lighted figures. With this electronic computer calculator I have been able to make two to three hundred or more calculations in one day, which ten years ago would have taken me many weeks. This is not nearly so miraculous as the response of my colon if there is anything within me that needs attention!

As a matter of fact, that is exactly what the human organism is, a mysterious, miraculous electronic computer administered by a tiny gland, the hypothalamus, located in the mid-brain. Nothing goes on in the human organism that is not watched over, controlled and administered by the hypothalamus.

Each chapter in this book indicates the relationship between the colon and a corresponding part of the human anatomy. Actually, after you have studied and absorbed the subject matter I have presented, you will be better able to understand your own anatomy as well as that of your child, and you may be much better able to cope with your own aches and pains, as well as with those of your children. This may even help you avoid the pitiful state of premature senility so prevalent today. Why so prevalent? Because people fail to understand the need to care for their miraculous organ, the colon. Each chapter in this book indicates what the relationship is between the colon and that part of the body indicated by the title. I have proved the material described and explained in the following pages to my own satisfaction — without any doubt or equivocation.

THE HYPOTHALAMUS

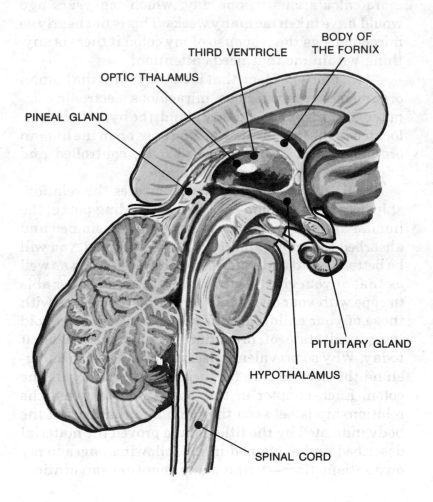

THIRD VENTRICLE

BODY OF THE FORNIX

OPTIC THALAMUS

PINEAL GLAND

PITUITARY GLAND

HYPOTHALAMUS

SPINAL CORD

CROSS SECTION OF THE LEFT SIDE OF THE BRAIN

Chapter 4.
The Hypothalamus:
The Control Center Of Your Body

No function or activity can take place without **energy**. This is true without any question or doubt when it concerns the human body. From the moment of conception, activity is in progress to enable the human fetus to grow. Upon birth and continuing on throughout the life of the body, nothing can take place without energy: the blood cannot be reorganized; the millions upon millions of red blood corpuscles—the hemoglobin — cannot be reproduced within the bones; the glands cannot create the hormones; the nerves and muscles cannot operate.

The hypothalamus, located in the middle of the brain, is in charge of distributing the proper amount of energy into the body. Up to the present day, comparatively little has been discovered of the vast scope of the administrating functions of the hypothalamus.

Looking at the accompanying illustration, we can see that the hypothalamus is not a gland, but a mere bundle of fibers, nerves, and blood vessels emanating from the thalamus, which is spread out on two sides of the space-like area known as the third ventricle. (The word ventricle means a cavity or chamber within an organ). Two branches of the thalamus are the metathalamus and the epithalamus, both of which are attached to the pineal gland. The hypothalamus structure forms the greater part of the floor of the third ventricle. It is enclosed somewhat like a capsule within the nerve fibers and the numerous nerve cells, **the connections of which are as yet not fully determined.**

Energy for the body's use does not just splash in haphazardly, without control and direction. Where does the energy for our body come from, and how is it distributed? It is difficult for the lay mind to grasp the fact that the primary energy which enables the glands to function and operate is that elusive cosmic force which is the basis of life and activity in everything in this universe.

What Are Cosmic Energy Vibrations?

The entire universe is composed of an infinite number of vibrations which, by their very condensed numbers, form matter, substance, or intangible things, much like the thousands of individual threads in a weaver's loom form a piece of cloth by the warp and woof — or crossing and re-crossing — of the threads. Cosmic energy vibrations are vibrations (or wave lengths) in the universe of inconceivably astronomical numbers per millimeter in length or per second in time.

Webster's Dictionary defines vibrations as the periodic motion of the particles of an elastic body or medium in alternately opposite directions from the position of perfect equilibrium, when that equilibrium has been disturbed. The word "cosmic" means "pertaining to the **cosmos**," a name which is synonymous with universe.

Webster gives quite an extensive definition of energy which I will sum up as, that which is the real existence of form, giving cause to life; power efficiently and forcefully exerted; the capacity for performing work.

By the above definitions, we are thus able to conclude that vibrations cause or form energy, and energy is the result of vibrations.

Man has been able to harness cosmic energy vibrations in many ways. One method is by an electric current generator which condenses the infinite number of vibrations into the almost insignificant volume of 60 cycles or vibrations per minute in the electric current in our homes, offices and shops.

Compare this 60 vibrations per **minute** in the electric wires of your home with the 49,390,000,000 vibrations per **second**, which is the number of cosmic energy vibrations of which a healthy male human body is composed! The healthy human female body is composed of only 20 million vibrations less than those of the male, namely 49,370,000,000 vibrations.

As the number of vibrations is so astronomical that it is apt to cause confusion in the mind of the un-initiated, a unit of 10 million vibrations per millimeter was established as the Angstrom Unit by Jonas Angstrom, astronomer and physicist, just over 100 years ago. This unit has greatly simplified the calculations of cosmic energy vibrations.

As a matter of fact, colors are a woven network of

vibrations with an infinite number of varieties of each color, depending on the number of vibrations existing above or below the number of vibrations present in the pure color.

On the basis of the Angstrom Unit, we find that the vibrations of the following pure colors are:

Violet	4,500 A.U.	Green	5,000 A.U.
Blue	4,750 A.U.	Yellow	6,000 A.U.
Orange	6,500 A.U.	Red	8,000 A.U.

Each of the various parts and glands of the human body has its own individual rate of cosmic energy vibrations, independent of the sum total of the body's composite vibrations. For example, the life of the individual is in the blood, specifically in the red blood corpuscles, or hemoglobin. We find that the hemoglobin in its healthy condition is composed of approximately 82,500 million vibrations per second. Correspondingly, the lung's vibrations are 67,250 million per second; the pituitary gland's vibrations are 58,000 million per second; the ear's vibrations are 47,750 million per second. Each part of the human anatomy has its own distinctive individual vibrations.

As ailments and sicknesses afflict the human body, its vibrations are correspondingly lowered or reduced, and when the ailing body has been healed of its afflictions, the vibrations return to their normal count and the individual feels strong and energetic.

With these few examples and explanations of cosmic energy vibrations, it should be easy to understand that a correct diagnostic system would be based on readings of such vibrations. When the body is sick,

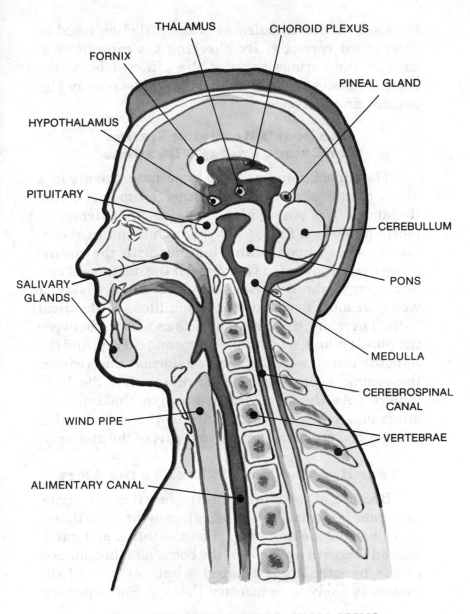

THALAMUS   CHOROID PLEXUS

FORNIX

PINEAL GLAND

HYPOTHALAMUS

PITUITARY

CEREBULLUM

SALIVARY
GLANDS

PONS

MEDULLA

CEREBROSPINAL
CANAL

WIND PIPE

VERTEBRAE

ALIMENTARY CANAL

THE HYPOTHALAMUS, THALAMUS
AND PINEAL GLAND

the kind, quality and degree of the affliction could be determined correctly. By checking the vibrations of each of the various parts of the afflicted body, the organ or gland actually involved could be readily pinpointed and corrected.

The Body's Receiving Station for Cosmic Energy Vibrations

The pineal gland and the hypothalamus are in a direct relationship with each other by means of the thalamus. The pineal gland acts as an antenna or receiving station for the body, which is in direct contact in some imponderable manner with the cosmic energy vibrations of the universe. If the full force of cosmic energy vibrations were received into the body, it would be more devastating than millions of electrical volts. Therefore, the thalamus acts as a buffer between the pineal gland, which collects cosmic energy, and the hypothalamus, which is the transformer that reduces the cosmic energy voltage down to what the body requires. As the transformer, the hypothalamus administers, regulates and controls the flow of this energy to every gland, organ and part of the anatomy.

Your Hypothalamus Is Ever on the Alert

Because of its administrative function, the hypothalamus is naturally very sensitive to the condition of every part of the anatomy. If fermentation and putrefaction starts in any part of the body, it is the function of the hypothalamus to alert whatever part of the system is likely to be affected thereby. Subsequently, the lymphatic stream is ordered to get busy and try to protect any part that may be affected.

To give an example, if a woman's colon is badly impacted or is afflicted by excessive fermentation in the area of the colon marked **mammary glands**, it is more than likely that the lymph glands in the area of the breast may collect waste matter, probably from the colon, and store it in the lymph glands of the breast, causing a lump to appear — as a warning. I have known such cases where the application of colon irrigations caused the lumps to disappear within a matter of days. The most important warnings of neglecting the colon are glandular disturbances.

It is not by accident that the very center of the transverse colon (see the *Colon Therapy Chart* for location) should be associated with the hypothalamus. It is at this point in the colon that the absorption of liquid and nutritious elements (which have already passed into the cecum and been propelled through the ascending colon) ceases, and straight-forward propulsion of waste matter and feces continues into the rectum. Impurities within the body have a definite effect on the mind and character; a putrid body reflects its condition in the level upon which the mind functions. Gross speech, behavior, and vulgarity are incompatible with a body that is clean within and without.

It is truly fantastic to attempt to evaluate the ramifications of the administrative functions of the hypothalamus. It may be a long time before science is able, even with the most sophisticated computer, to work these imponderable problems into mathematical fig-

THE PITUITARY GLAND

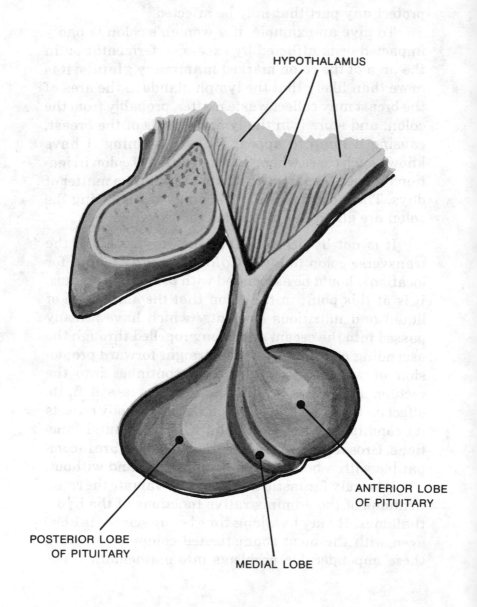

HYPOTHALAMUS

ANTERIOR LOBE
OF PITUITARY

POSTERIOR LOBE
OF PITUITARY

MEDIAL LOBE

ures. Even our thoughts are more or less subject to the functions of the hypothalamus.

Considering the physical fact that nerves spread out to every part of the brain from the hypothalamus, and that the cleaner the body is, the higher the cosmic energy vibrations available to the brain, it certainly pays to cleanse the body and keep the colon in a constantly clean and healthy condition.

Pituitary Gland — Neighbor to the Hypothalamus

A glance at the illustration of the **normal** colon (located in the front of the book) will reveal to you the shape of a healthy colon. Unfortunately, we are only likely to find this perfect outline in the colon of a tiny infant before the wrong kind of food has had the opportunity to distort it. This is the shape originated by our Creator. Man, being a **free moral agent**, has consistently corrupted the foods and beverages which he has ingested, resulting in fantastic distortions of the colon as he grows older. The colon does not become afflicted overnight. Every time waste matter accumulates in the colon, which results in fermentation and putrefaction, a disturbance takes place both in the afflicted area of the colon and in its corresponding part of the anatomy. The afflicted areas of the anatomy are shown in relationship to the various sacculations of the colon on the *Colon Therapy Chart*.

The colon begins on your right hand side in or just above the groin, in the pelvis. The first pouch, which you will see on the left side of the picture and at the bot-

THE CECUM

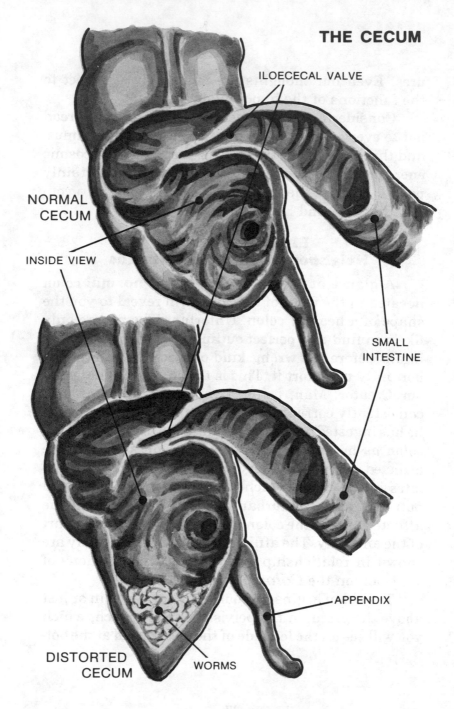

ILOECECAL VALVE

NORMAL CECUM

INSIDE VIEW

SMALL INTESTINE

DISTORTED CECUM

WORMS

APPENDIX

tom of the ascending colon, is called the cecum. At the very center of the bottom of this pouch you will see the word **pituitary**. This means that the pituitary gland (located in the brain) and this area of the colon have an electronic, vibratory relationship.

When an X ray of the colon shows this pouch to be in the form of a "V," illustrated in the sketch which accompanies this chapter, one can be sure that a group of worms has colonized in this particular location. I have usually found that these turn out to be tape worms. This affliction of the cecum pouch of the colon usually results in the development of a state of constant fatigue.

The pituitary gland, as you will notice from the illustration, is composed of three general sections: the posterior lobe, also known as the pars nervosa, indicating its particular association with the nerve system of the body; the anterior lobe, also referred to as the pars glandularis or glandular part; and the medial lobe, which consists of a strip between the other two lobes.

The three lobes of the pituitary gland are directly affected by any serious disturbance in this region of the cecum. The posterior pituitary, having direct nerve connections with the brain, is involved in virtually every activity of the body, so that anything irregular in this location in the cecum has repercussions in many unsuspected ways.

Consider the temperature of the body, which the posterior pituitary in many ways controls. When the weather is hot, the pores of the skin open and allow perspiration to take place, while in cold weather the pores are closed to retain heat in the body and prevent evaporation. The posterior pituitary also involves the regulation of water in the system. The body is composed of between 75% and 80% distilled water which is essential for the flow of the lymph stream. This stream of water collects impurities throughout the body which eventually are passed both through the kidneys and into the colon. One type of cecum disturbance may cause excessive liquids in the colon, resulting in diarrhea, another may inhibit water from getting into the colon, causing constipation to be dry and painful. Thus, we have a close relationship between the posterior pituitary and the cecum. The anterior pituitary, on the other hand, is involved in the functions of the glands, generating hormones for the reproductive organs, the adrenal glands, the thyroid, the liver and for the pancreas. Each of these will be discussed in their respective chapters in due sequence. It is clearly evident how a disturbance of this area of the cecum has a great many ramifications.

In my book *Become Younger*, I have given the case of a young man who went through all the agonies of military injections, and as a result was debilitated and weakened. Medications aggravated his condition and he was released because of is disability, although upon induction he was found to be in excellent condition. When he came to us, he was directed to have an X ray of his colon which revealed the typical worm-nest outline of the cecum. He passed stacks of worms and improved. One may read this account in *Become Younger*.

Very few people realize how directly the condition of the colon is related to weariness, and particularly to stress and nervousness. Before the danger point is reached in these insidious disturbances, the colon frequently tries to give warning signals, sometimes in the form of cramps, but usually in the form of more or less severe constipation discomforts. They never assail humans "out of the blue," and when the limit of tolerance is just about reached, the trouble is triggered by events such as the death of a loved one or family disruption, such as divorce or separation. Personal injury, loss of work, or financial troubles may be contributing factors, or perhaps any of three or four dozen other personal calamities. It is almost impossible to maintain a clear mind and proper mental and spiritual equilibrium when we allow the colon to go unattended for too long a time. The relationship of the pituitary gland to the cecum, as well as to the functions of the body as a whole, is too intimately involved to be overlooked.

We have found that colon irrigations can, and do, prevent far more distress than people realize. It is not enough to take just one or two colonics, then quit. One should take as many as are necessary to leave the colon perfectly clean. Once the colon has been thoroughly washed, at least two irrigations should be taken twice a year, throughout life — yes, as long as we live. Prevention is much better than cure, particularly to avoid premature senility!

Chapter 5.
Keeping A Clear Head

Your Eyes

Between the ileo-cecal valve in the colon and the juncture of the next sacculation above it, we have the area which reflects the relationship to the **eyes**. Here we have another very delicate situation. The optic system is indeed a miracle to contemplate.

It is a sin and a crime the way people take their eyes and their vision for granted — until their eyesight becomes dim or they go blind. This area, perhaps more than any other, should have first consideration.

Actually our optic system is far too complicated to be described intelligently in such a brief dissertation. In the first place, the eyes are merely contributing factors in our visual perception of things seen. Somewhat like our ears, cosmic energy vibrations are the means by which forms and color are transmitted to the brain for the interpretation that we spell out in the words, "I see."

The first step in our vision involves the retina, which is the delicate membrane of the eye representing the end, or terminal expansion, of the optic nerve. As thin as the retina is, it is composed of several layers, among which are the pigment layers that first register color, then the nerve layer, followed by about seven other layers which all comprise the retina. The state and condition of each one of these layers reflects on the kind, quality and degree of vision just like the setting on the lens of a complicated photographic camera.

In the first layer of the retina there are "rods" and "cones" which transmit the vibrations of the object in the form of messages to the nerve cells, to the chiasm or x-crossing, ending in the brain at the thalamus and the third ventricle. The third ventricle is a very important open space inside the temple, extending between the optic thalamus and the brain. (See accompanying illustration of the hypothalamus.)

To clarify the presence of the rods and cones in the retina, you should know that there are altogether only about 125,000,000 (that's right, 125 million) rods and cones, besides about 1,250,000 fibers in the optic nerve. One would almost be justified in considering that with these figures we would have a wide margin of safety with our retina in particular, and in our vision generally; but remember that these infinitesimal, microscopic, wee objects require two very essential things in order to serve you with vision: they need nutrition and cleanliness. They need ample, natural, nutritional food and clean excretory channels for the removal of toxic waste from the body. With the brief time and space at our disposal here, it would be too great a task to describe the paths that the object you are looking at must take to be transmitted accurately to the brain, so you may correctly understand and interpret what you see. In other words, the shapes, forms, colors and perspectives of objects within the range of your vision are carried by vibration impulses through the respective maze

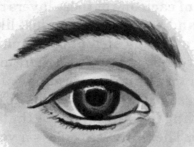

The Right Eye of a Healthy Young Woman
Alert When Awake . . .

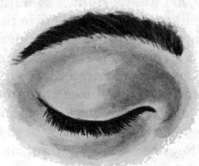

Relaxed When Asleep

"Do not envy good health, build up your own."

N.W. Walker

THE EYE

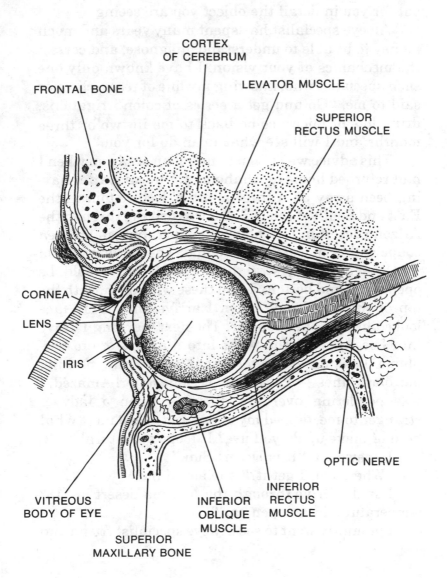

CORTEX
OF CEREBRUM

FRONTAL BONE

LEVATOR MUSCLE

SUPERIOR
RECTUS MUSCLE

CORNEA

LENS

IRIS

OPTIC NERVE

VITREOUS
BODY OF EYE

INFERIOR
OBLIQUE
MUSCLE

INFERIOR
RECTUS
MUSCLE

SUPERIOR
MAXILLARY BONE

of nerves which correspond to each item, all of these co-ordinating in the brain, so that the brain will spell out for you in detail the object you are seeing.

An eye specialist has spent many years and much money to be able to understand, diagnose, and correct the mechanics of your vision. I have known only one such specialist who, knowing my line of research, once said to me, "Go and get a series of colon irrigations, drink lots of juices, come back to me in two or three months and I will see what I can do for you."

This advice was given to me on an occasion when I had returned home to Ahaheim, California, after having been away on a three months' lecture tour in the East and South of the U.S.A. I was driving through the Arizona desert in 118° blazing temperature, in an open coupe with a house trailer behind. The car windshield was the old type, straight across, which could be opened top and bottom. I had these wide open, with the top of the car down. When I arrived home my face looked like a boiled lobster. The next morning I drove into Los Angeles and went into a drug store to telephone. Looking at the telephone book I saw nothing but black lines — I could not see one letter! Amazed, I was pondering over my dilemma when a lady, a stranger to me, tapped my elbow and asked me, "What kind of make-up do you use? It looks so natural."

I answered, "It is Desert Sun."

"Where can I get it?" she asked me.

I said, "Drive through the Arizona desert in 118° temperature, in an open car!"

I promptly went to see my eye specialist friend and

subsequently followed his advice. For three weeks I had three colon irrigations a week and drank, besides my other juices and salads, two pints daily of the combination of carrot-celery-parsley-and-endive juice. I went to him again before the month was over, and he thought it was a miracle! He fitted me with glasses which I used for about four or five weeks for reading only. One day in the car I accidentally sat on them and never had them replaced.

Neither the juices nor the colon irrigations alone, one without the other, could have been as effective as combining the two.

I should mention here the damage which could be done to the optic system by the inorganic mineral elements in water. These elements cannot be assimilated constructively by the human body. The body *does* need mineral elements, but these must be obtained from vegetation in which the inorganic elements of the soil are converted into life-containing, nourishing food. A person drinking one or two pints of regular well, spring or faucet water daily would, in about 40 years time, have between 200 and 300 pounds of lime pass through his body. Fortunately, most of this is eliminated, but some is bound to remain. Depending on what part of the body this remnant settles in, sooner or later trouble will develop in that part. Far too many heart attacks could be blamed on such inorganic elements clogging up the blood vessels. Many varicose veins could be found to blame their condition on these inorganic mineral elements as the contributing factor. The optic system is not less liable to be so afflicted. The answer is

47

simply to use only water which has been steam-distilled. My book, **Water Can Undermine Your Health**, will give you the information you need to be safeguarded from this danger. Of course fresh, raw vegetable and fruit juices are composed of pure, naturally distilled water. In fact, bear in mind that the human body is composed of between 75% and 80% **distilled water**.

Nearly everyone with good vision takes their eyes for granted. That is a great mistake. When we neglect to care for our eyes, we lay ourselves wide open to future trouble. The problem is, people cannot imagine themselves as being unable to see! Nearly every elderly person whose vision is dim could tell you a tale of woe because they did not give their eyes the attention they required. At the same time, never for one moment lose sight of the fact that the colon, all too often, is a contributing factor in eye trouble.

I had a friend in New York years ago, a retired Captain in the Scottish Highlanders, in his 50's, whose vision in Britain had been perfect. When in this country, not realizing how harmful they are, he learned to indulge in the commonly used American processed and fried foods. He became badly constipated, a condition which never afflicted him at home in Scotland. One day he complained to me that he was having trouble with his eyes, and he said to me, "I wonder if having to strain as I do, at stool, because of this confounded constipation, could have effected my eyes?" I told him undoubtedly that this was one contributing factor which could cause trouble with the retina. When he consulted a good eye specialist this was confirmed.

Never underestimate the value of a clean colon. Think ahead. Do all you possibly can to avoid dimness of your eyes and premature senility.

Ears and Ear Trouble

Proceeding upward on the diagram of the colon, past the ileo-cecal valve, we come to a particularly sensitive area which is **electronically related** to the area of the brain which controls the **ears** — the auditory or acoustic system.

It should be understood that the relationship between the sacculations of the colon and the various organs and glands (or parts of the body remotely located from the colon) does not necessarily involve a drastic affliction, although such a situation does occur occasionally. Such a relationship, which may manifest itself at the time of maximum fermentation or putrefaction in the colon, may simply develop into a warning signal.

For example, an ulcer may develop in this particular sacculation of the colon, and this irritation may disturb the sensitive auditory system. The common practice, when the irritation is sufficiently annoying, is to consult an "ear specialist." If he does not correct the trouble, it worsens. On the other hand, being familiar with **colon therapy**, we would first take a series of colon irrigations. We have found that the outcome of this method is often a complete disappearance of the ear trouble, sometimes within a matter of hours. This would prove to us that the ear irritation was a signal to

THE EAR

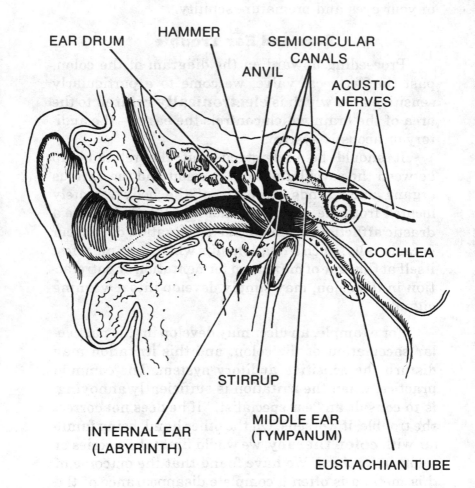

EAR DRUM

HAMMER

ANVIL

SEMICIRCULAR
CANALS

ACUSTIC
NERVES

COCHLEA

STIRRUP

MIDDLE EAR
(TYMPANUM)

INTERNAL EAR
(LABYRINTH)

EUSTACHIAN TUBE

clean house within. It has been cumulative, satisfactory results like this that has urged us on to deeper and deeper research.

Of course we must always be conscious of the relationships existing between the scattered glands in our system. The function of the auditory system is under the administration of the hypothalamus in the midbrain which, in turn, functions through the pituitary gland. Obviously, it requires a vast knowledge of the entire human anatomy and the entire system of related and inter-related functions and activities of the many parts of the body to make a satisfactory diagnosis.

We can be sure that we can never go wrong when we start from the very beginning with high enemas and colon irrigations. If the body from infancy has been brought up and nourished as was originally intended, and meticulous attention paid to the elimination of waste matter, there should be no ailments or bodily discomforts. Our trouble is **civilization** which has become addicted to indoctrination, salesmanship, and wrong thinking. Of course, as we cannot see inside the body, there are times when an X ray is of inestimable help to determine from the condition of the colon what needs to be corrected, and in the order of importance.

I use the word "electronic" in reference to the relation and inter-relation of the colon with other parts of the body, in a descriptive sense. Electronics is that branch of physics which treats with the emission, behavior and effects of electrons. Electrons are components of atoms. As we have learned on radio and televi-

THE EAR

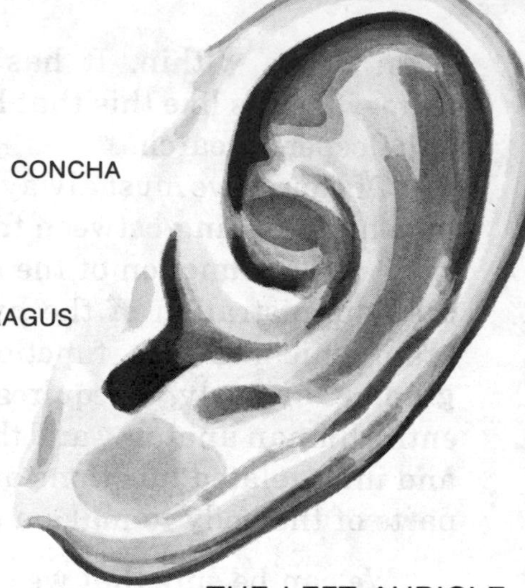

CONCHA

TRAGUS

THE LEFT AURICLE
AND CONCHA

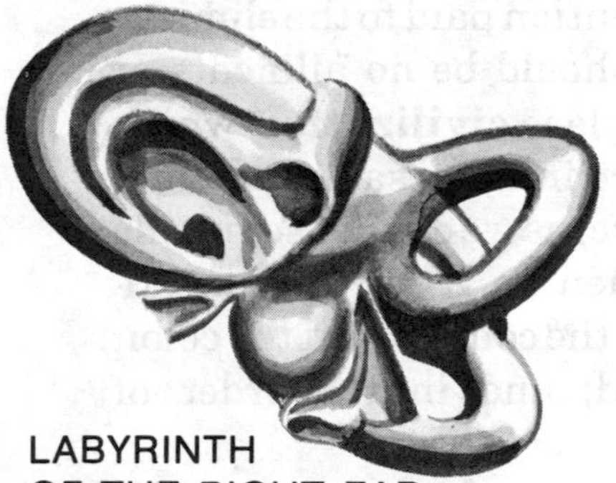

UPPER LIGAMENT
OF THE MALLET

MALLET OR
HAMMER

LABYRINTH
OF THE RIGHT EAR
WITH THE INTERNAL
AUDITORY PASSAGE,
AQUEDUCT OF THE
VESTIBULE, AND AQUEDUCT
OF THE COCHLEA

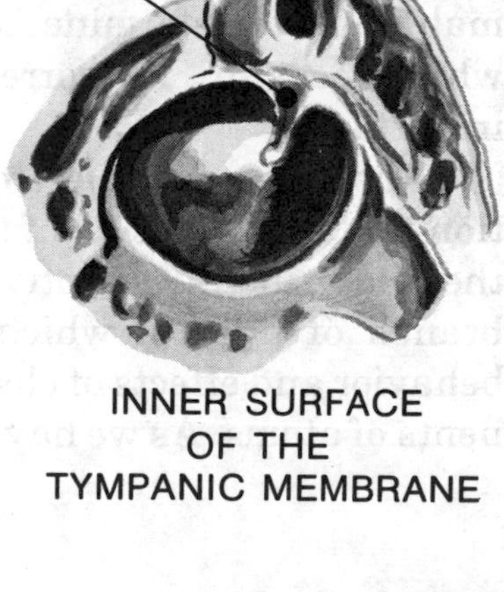

INNER SURFACE
OF THE
TYMPANIC MEMBRANE

sion, these electrons emit cosmic energy vibrations that stagger the imagination. It is just by means of these cosmic energy vibrations that the hypothalamus is able to administer, control, and otherwise influence virtually every function and activity of the infinite number of areas, spots and points throughout the body and, in turn, everything connected with them. Tenuous as these vibrations are, they nevertheless are there for our use and understanding.

Our hearing apparatus is far more wonderful than any contraption man has ever devised. The organ of hearing is composed of the external ear, which is visible, the middle ear known as the tympanum, and the internal ear called the labyrinth. The outer ear is composed of an expansion of the skin structure and the external auditory canal through which sound wave vibrations enter. The middle ear is composed of the tympanum, which is the Latin word meaning "drum," commonly called the eardrum. Here are also "ear bones" which are far more sensitive than a tuning fork. We also have the Eustachian tube connecting with the pharynx, which is a sensitive membrane situated back of the nose, mouth and larynx, and extends to the base of the skull opposite the sixth cervical vertebra of the spine.

By means of the tympanic membrane, sound vibrations are transmitted to the cochlea of the internal ear. Cochlea is derived from the Greek word "kochlos," which means "conch shell." The cochlea resembles a snail shell; the tube in the cochlea makes 2½ turns forming a spiral canal, 1½ inches long from end to end.

The central, closed end of the canal registers low tones or vibrations expressed by the base cleff sign 𝄢 in music, while the outer extension registers the high tones or vibrations, expressed by the treble cleff sign 𝄞 in music.

You can certainly understand my brief dissertation on the hearing problem, how delicate and far reaching it is. We do not hear with our ears; they merely transmit sounds to the brain, and the brain translates them for our understanding. Any interference along the line affects the quality of our ability to hear. The colon is intimately involved somewhere along the line.

I hope this little synopsis I have tried to give you will suffice to make you conscious of the intricacy of your hearing apparatus. I can only leave it for your intelligence to perceive the need to keep the inside of your body as clean as you possibly can, so that it may serve you well and efficiently for the rest of your life.

Nasal Catarrh and Asthma

Moving farther along on our trip up the right side of the ascending colon, we come to two related afflictions, namely **nasal catarrh** and **asthma**. These can be discussed together because they are both derivatives of the same cause. Whatever causes excess mucus to form in the upper regions of the system can be counted upon to start a mucous chain-reaction.

Frequently, the first symptoms to appear when mucus begins to accumulate is the feeling of a draft which may cause one to sneeze. The usual response to this is, "I'm catching a cold!" Let me set your mind at ease. We are not able to "catch a cold." It is the cold that catches us! The unhealthy mucus that we have generated has a magnetic attraction for a cooler temperature, causing the organs involved with the mucus to afflict the victim. This affliction may strike at the nose or at the throat and frequently the lungs.

I could fill volumes with instances where human beings, from babies to tottering seniles, changed their eating and drinking habits and saw their colds, hay fever, asthma and other mucus afflictions completely disappear after having colon irrigations.

For example, in my book *Become Younger*, read about the precious old lady who banished her own mucus afflictions, then years later sent her daughter, who was strictly medical-minded, off for a three weeks' vacation so that Grandma could take care of the little two-year-old boy. The poor little fellow had not been able to get a good night's sleep since shortly after he was born, when he was put on cow's milk and the "scientific" formulas for babies. Just as soon as the daughter was out of the way, Grandma gave the baby an enema and fed him orange juice. The first night on this program the little fellow slept soundly from 8 p.m. to 6 a.m. But you may read the account for yourself.

For many years scientists and researchers have been climbing up one side of the rainbow and down the other in their well-financed search for the elusive germ, bug, virus or what have you, that could be blamed for **causing** colds and analogous mucous ailments. To this day, they are still pursuing that fading, useless chase. The **cause** of these annoying disturbances is of course **mucus**. Eliminate whatever causes mucus to form, as in colds, asthma, bronchitis, and the like, and no colds can be experienced.

I was greatly amused when, sometime in the 1920's, certain scientists caused their hobby to make the headlines by declaring that they had discovered a "germ" which was definitely responsible for the common cold, **but** that it was too small and elusive to be caught and (note this) too small to be seen by their most powerful microscopes. Nevertheless, they "discovered" such a germ.

During the past four-score years we have seen far too many colds and analogous ailments disappear by removing cow's milk and other mucous-forming foods from the diet and cleansing the body with high enemas and colon irrigations.

Bear in mind, please, that it would take some 12, 15, or more enemas to get the results which can be obtained by each properly administered colon irrigation. The pathway of the scientists, in my experience, leads to by-passing a colon irrigation. This is not good, as colon irrigations are invariably effective.

I would like to quote from my book *Fresh Vegetable & Fruit Juices*, in which you will read, "... since 1946, according to word I have from England, some scientists under the $150,000 a year patronage of the British Government's "Medical Research Council" have been hunting — and, you know, the British are notorious for their hunting — for a **cold bug**, **germ**, or **virus** as the culprit which could be accused of being responsible for the generation of the **common cold**." I

56

am sure that you will thoroughly enjoy reading this whole account. It is too ludicrous for comment.

I am utterly amazed that an orthodox practitioner rarely considers it worthwhile to look to the colon for the banishment of the affliction. If they only will do so, they will understand the carpenter who sent a post card to Sears Roebuck asking, "Where is that saw I ordered and paid for a month ago?" Then he added a postscript: "Excuse me. I just found the saw under my bench." Colds and their analogous ailments are Nature's very effective way to warn us to get busy and do some housecleaning inside our body.

I have referred to milk as being the most mucous-forming food we can use. Raw milk would be bad enough, but to pasteurize or homogenize it is worse. Besides milk, processed cheeses are the frequent cause of excessive mucus. Devitalized starches and sugar are both mucus culprits and when removed from the diet the beneficial results are perceptive. Above all, invariably start with cleansing the colon.

Ascorbic acid (Vitamin C) is depleted in the body when it is called upon to fight colds for you; replenish the body with this valuable element and see how your cold will completely disappear. Read and study the chapter entitled **Connective Tissue and Vitamin C** in this book. This is important. The cold it may banish may be **yours!**

Hay Fever

We will now move over to the other side of the cecum to the spot directly opposite the ileo-cecal valve.

This spot, you will notice, is marked **hay fever**. It is quite significant that the spot should occur facing the flow of residue from the small intestine into the colon. This residue is composed of the undigested food which by-passed the absorption of nutrients from the digested food through the walls of the small intestine. Normally, most of the contents of this residue is converted into feces and, in due course, is propelled through the five feet of large intestine (the colon) for evacuation.

Few people, however, have such a "normal" residue, which can only be the result of proper and correct nutrition. Rarely do people eat the right kinds of food for the attainment of health. This is consequently the starting point for the manufacture of **hay fever**. I suppose it seems strange to ascribe the running nose, the throat trouble and all the concomitant hay fever symptoms to the contents and the condition of the colon, but this is only strange to those who have not seen hay fever disappear after a series of colon irrigations. We have seen scores of them! If this procedure of cleansing the colon was to be successful in one or two instances and no more, then there would be justifiable doubts, but seeing this happen consistently over and over again — well, what would **your** answer be?

What triggers the building-up of the mucous condition which manifests itself in what people call hay fever? It can only be the result of what has been taken into the system. Pollen does not cause hay fever; if it did, then everybody sniffing pollen would have hay fever and that is not the case. I have sniffed every kind of pollen and I do not yet know what hay fever feels like.

The troublesome element in hay fever is the copious amount of mucus which accompanies it. There are two kinds of mucus. There is the lubricating mucus in the mucosa, or lubricating system, which is natural and necessary in every human body. Then, there is the pathogenic mucus that is the result of eating and drinking certain foods. This pathogenic mucus is the ideal media for propagating germs, microbes, and bacteria. Cow's milk is the most prolific source of this type of mucus. That is why a baby raised mostly on cow's milk has a constantly running nose. That is why so many young people drinking cow's milk are afflicted with colds and infected tonsils, not to mention pimples, which are mucus turned into pus that the body tries to excrete through the skin. I would consider it very strange if these troubles and discomforts were to persist after the afflicted person has avoided cow's milk and taken a series of colon irrigations. To date, after scores of years of research and observation, I have yet to find a single instance of such an irrigation failing to be effective when cow's milk has been discarded. Naturally, if such a victim gets rid of these afflictions by this natural means mentioned above but continues to eat and drink what caused the trouble in the first place, he most assuredly must expect a recurrence of his troubles.

Admittedly, it is not an easy matter to change one's diet, particularly when the taste buds have been perverted for a lifetime. Therefore, one must begin to train the **willpower** and administer to oneself drastic discipline. Unfortunately, few people are willing or mentally equipped to do this, but, in the final analysis, is it not much better to undergo hard, nutritional training in the present, rather than have to look forward to a premature senility with all its concomitant discomforts to self and others?

This is not the time or place for me to give a program of diet which could build up the system and give the individual the opportunity to live longer, more abundantly, and with a better degree of health than he previously experienced when he ate all kinds of processed, fried, and over-cooked foods. I recommend that you obtain my book *A Guide to Diet & Salads*, which is used by people the world over as a guide to better nutrition.

Every X ray of hay fever victims that I have seen has invariably shown trouble in this particular spot which you will see marked on the left hand side of my *Colon Therapy Chart*. This 17" x 22" wall chart has been reduced and reproduced in this book for your easy reference.

If you have never had a colon irrigation you have missed the most pleasant and comfortable means by which the colon can be washed out. You are able to lie restfully on the colonic table for a half, to one hour, depending on the condition of your colon.

Look in the classified telephone directory for *Chiropractors, Naturopaths, Physiotherapists* and ask if they have colonic equipment, or look under *Colonics* or *Colon Irrigations*.

Colon irrigations are of such immeasurable value in our domestic economy that everybody should make it a practice to have them once or twice a year as long as they live. I am convinced that by this means the life expectancy can be lengthened considerably.

Don't fail to study **Connective Tissue and Vitamin C**, the final chapter in this book! The **hay fever it banishes may be yours!**

Tonsils: Should We Keep Them?

Next, further up on this side of the cecum, we find that the middle of the pouch or sacculation is labeled **tonsils**. This is to indicate that this area has some relationship with the glands in the throat known as tonsils.

Did anyone ever tell you that tonsils have no useful purpose, and that they should be removed during childhood in order to prevent their having to be taken out later in life? Those who ascribe this theory do not know what they are talking about.

My medical dictionary brushes off the subject by merely stating that, "The tonsil is a small almond-shaped body situated on each side, between the front and the rear pillars, of the soft palate. It consists of an aggregation of from 10 to 18 small follicles (bags or crypts) covered by a mucous membrane." The entire healing profession has greatly minimized the vital importance of these two indispensable glands, the tonsils.

It is true that Almighty God made man out of the dust of the earth, in His own image, and when He breathed into him the breath of life, man became a living soul, and it was good. God never placed in the human body anything that was not useful and necessary. So, like every other gland in the body, the tonsils have their part in the economy of the human anatomy, its functions and activities.

THE PHARYNGEAL CAVITY
SEEN FROM BEHIND

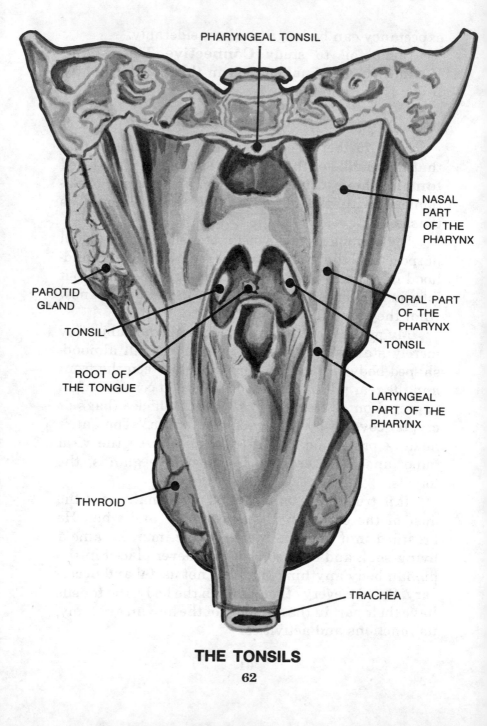

PHARYNGEAL TONSIL

NASAL PART OF THE PHARYNX

PAROTID GLAND

ORAL PART OF THE PHARYNX

TONSIL

TONSIL

ROOT OF THE TONGUE

LARYNGEAL PART OF THE PHARYNX

THYROID

TRACHEA

THE TONSILS

I have studied very carefully many of the books published by the brothers I. and G. Calderoli of Bergamo, Italy, recounting in detail the results of their 30 years of intensive research on tonsils, in the Universities of Vienna and Berlin. I have many of their books, written in Italian, and refer to them often. When I met Dr. Guido Calderoli in Bergamo, Italy some years ago, we discussed this subject very thoroughly. I asked him if any of the patients suffering with tonsils happened to be bothered with aches or pains in the right side, under the ribs. He never paid much attention to this, but as he thought back, he remembered it was a frequent complaint which was often attributed to some disturbance in the appendix. I asked if any of his patients had an appendectomy after the tonsils had been "taken care of." He did not remember any instance where this took place, and he agreed that undoubtedly the clearing up of the tonsil ailment may have indirectly had something to do with the colon.

Some people assume the most important function of the tonsils is to collect germs, microbes and bacteria, preventing their entrance into the system. Such statements come from those who either are not aware that the body is literally filled with conflicting germs or do not know the deeper activities of the glands in the body. Swollen tonsils are among the most notorious afflictions of children and young people, purely and simply because they neglect to respond to the call of their bowels and fail to understand the importance of proper nutrition. Adults are just as prone to neglect these two basic principles in the attainment and the maintenance of health. Without having studied the reason why Almighty God placed the tonsils where they are, nor investigated the after-effects of removing afflicted tonsils, the general custom for generations has been to cut them out.

Unquestionably, there is an endocrine gland correlation between tonsils, reproductive organs, and the cecum pouch of the colon. Man cannot interfere with this intimate relationship without grave danger.

Let me give you a vivid example which definitely related the cecum to a tonsil affliction. I had a friend in New York who had a beautiful little home out on the Island. She kept her home meticulously clean and in order, and she spent much of her spare time in the maintenance of her garden, which had beautiful roses and other flowers.

I met her one day on 42nd Street in New York as I was on my way to Grand Central Station. I naturally asked how she was. She told me that for nearly two weeks she had suffered with a persistent sore throat. Catherine, a nurse and co-worker in her office, had urged her to go to the hospital without delay and have her tonsils removed. I strongly protested and recommended that she have a series of colon irrigations. She objected to this, saying that after her recovery from the tonsillectomy she was planning on taking Catherine's advice to have an appendectomy, as she had a pain on her right side below her ribs. Again I protested, to which she replied, "I would have you know that Catherine was head of one of the largest hospital's nursing divisions for 20 years. Who are you to know more than she?"

My final words to her were, "My dear lady, I have given you my advice. If you go through with your tonsillectomy you will regret it for the rest of your life." I did not see this lady again until nearly one year later when we happened to meet almost at the same spot on 42nd Street. She was the one who stopped me. I did not recognize her. I asked how her house on the Island with all her beautiful flowers was coming along. "Oh," she said, "I had to sell that six months ago. It was too much for me to keep up. I now have a small apartment where I can go home at lunch time and relax, and when I get through at the office I go home and rest for the remainder of the day." I asked if she had gone through with the appendectomy, and she said her appendix trouble did not develop after her tonsillectomy, so she did nothing about it.

A young doctor, only 38 years of age, whose tonsils were removed declared, "I myself feel a progressive weariness. I am always tired, even after resting."

A 25-year-old young woman had only one tonsil removed when she was 21 years old; nevertheless, after her tonsillectomy she began to take notice of disturbances which had never afflicted her before. She had pains in her back; she frequently perspired, her hands were always moist; she had frequent attacks of dizziness, and if meals were late she felt faint. She also experienced restlessness in sleep with morning fatigue, and general physical weakness. She found herself sloven in her housekeeping, and she never felt like singing anymore.

A 28-year-old electrical technician, ten years after

tonsil removal, declared, "I must have been born tired. My family and friends ridicule me."

An examination of thousands of workmen whose tonsils were removed in their youth clearly demonstrated the afflictions following a tonsillectomy — loss of physical, sexual and mental dynamism.

In the year 1952, England imported from Italy many hundreds of mine workers. Why? Because some 60% of the British youth were without tonsils and consequently constantly too tired for this kind of work. Italy, having the lowest percentage in Europe of tonsillectomies, had men who were virile and vigorous. Thirty years of study in Italy proved that, sooner or later, tonsillectomies reduced vigor and vitality in its victims.

The two Calderoli brothers spent 30 years in deep research on the subject, and this is a long enough time to arrive at many undeniable conclusions. Their conclusions resulted from innumerable studies of victims of tonsillectomies. These studies revealed that young women who were formerly normal in their affection and attraction for young men gradually had their feelings reversed, no longer wanting to have anything to do with them. Wives who formerly were a closely-knit, loving and an attentive member of their family, carefully solicitous of their children, husband and other members of the family, found themselves annoyed with the children, paid little or no attention to their needs and habits, neglected their household duties, and generally become slovenly.

Businessmen whose tonsils were afflicted and removed in their adulthood became lax in business, lost interest in their social contacts and experienced unbearable fatigue. With thirty years of consistent proof of this state of affairs, it is evident to me that my own experiences with people simply followed this natural pattern.

Tonsils have a definite relation to the sex or reproductive organs, called the gonads (the testicles and the ovaries). The Calderolis proved that men and women who are 28 years old and less and without tonsils are less masculine and less feminine, respectively.

Extended physiological and clinical research has revealed that there is an intimate relationship between tonsils and ovaries. The removal of tonsils can readily affect the frequency and volume of menstruation, a fact which should alert women to alarm. In such cases, leucorrhea between periods of menstruation frequently becomes a serious problem. Many a mother has panicked at her daughter's leucorrhea, and also at the excessive loss of blood during menstruation.

As I have already tried to emphasize, the loss of sex sensitivity in young women frequently follows the removal of tonsils. They become frigid. Many were asked: "Why then did you get married?" They answered, "Because everybody does. Besides, it establishes me." The ultimate end of such marriages is divorce or even worse calamities. Such women lose their ability to enjoy life and to sustain the interest and the spirit of the man and of the family.

At the time Dr. Calderoli wrote his book, *Popoli Senza Tonsille (People Without Tonsils)*, there were three large institutions in Italy for young women. They all refused admission to women whose tonsils had been removed. The deans of these institutions gave as their reason: "Generally, with their tonsils removed they are lazy, their character has changed as a result of the tonsillectomy, and their outlook on life has degenerated."

It is an indisputable matter of fact that Almighty God did not plan for mediocrity but rather the development of true masculinity and true femininity, because only by this means can the specie be perpetuated. A tonsillectomy is, therefore, a degrading practice not only affecting the individual, but likewise the family, the race and society, contributing to the decadence of the specie.

The eventual result of tonsil removal has been reduced activity and cheerfulness in children, less buoyancy in young people, and general lassitude in adults. Weariness is noticeable in students, in married life, in the family and in social activities. Young women deprived of their tonsils are likely to lose their inclination towards normal sex conduct and develop an aversion to maternity. The famous Doctors Calderoli have proved beyond a doubt that tonsils are so essential in the life of the individual that their extirpation, their removal, can have frustrating, devastating effects and repercussions for the rest of the individual's life.

In past generations, and to this very day, tonsils were considered organs of defense and of protection. Their function was considered limited to, and circumscribed by, the trapping and catching of germs and microbes passing through the nose and mouth. If that were an infallible fact, then everybody — **everybody** — would be afflicted with whatever happens to be the prevailing ailment. But that is not the case. It is the condition of the system, as exemplified by what is taking place in the colon, that can make the tonsils give their warnings.

The tonsils and the condition of the colon must **always** be considered and linked as warning factors. Apart from the importance of the tonsils themselves, there are clear, distinct, explicit reasons for giving meticulous attention to the colon. No one else can be responsible for your colon; it is **your** responsibility. I consider colon irrigations to be the most vital phase of the care of the body. The removal of offending waste matter from the colon automatically removes or reduces the obstruction from the throat, the nasal cavities and wherever the trouble with the tonsils has its inception.

Research has proved that tonsil removal is having serious consequences and great repercussions in the civil life of nations. Considering national statistics, it is not surprising to learn that about one third of the married people in the United States of America, in Europe and in the Scandinavian countries have no children, one third with only one. This, in fact, could be due to the aftermath of wholesale tonsillectomies.

I personally, in my own direct contact with people, have never known it to fail that when the tonsils are afflicted, enemas and colon irrigations cleared them up.

As this manuscript is about to go to press, I have just received a letter from a lady in Kansas, from which

I extract the following:

"We have two children ages six and seven. Our seven year old is excellent at spelling. . . . our six-year-old boy needs all the help he can get. He had to have his tonsils out when he was four years old, and when that was over we had one problem after another. They now say that he is mentally retarded and has a very severe learning disability. I want to do anything possible to help my son. He is a year behind what he should be, but he is really a bright child. I just know the Lord will completely deliver him. He was normal in every way before having his tonsils removed. We have hit a dead end finding out what happened to our son. He has seen every kind of doctor possible and still no answer. Please, if you can help me, tell me how and where. Thanking you for your great work — Praise the Lord."

Signed: Mrs. Smith

What About a Sore Throat?

A sore throat can be caused by any one or more of many reasons, causes and circumstances. In the first place, the mouth is the principal organ through which anything can enter the human system. The one thing we do regularly, every minute of the day and night, is to breathe. What do we breathe? We naturally breathe the air which happens to be in the atmosphere in which we

70

find ourselves. While air is composed of nitrogen and oxygen, in this day and generation we are virtually encased in an aura of pollution, not the least of which are the myriads and myriads of germs, viruses and bacteria which we cannot see. The throat is equipped with protective devices which prevent such parasites from entering the body — to a certain extent. If the body is pure and thoroughly clean, germs, virus and bacteria cannot exist in it, because these parasites are scavengers created for the specific purpose of destroying putrefactive waste matter, wherever it may happen to be. If the body is free of such waste matter there is nothing for these scavengers to feed on, and where there is no life-sustaining material, life perishes. Consequently, if a sore throat develops, where can the soreness come from? It is the natural result of the irritation of parasites rummaging in the region of the throat, and a warning to proceed with a body-cleansing as quickly as possible. When the throat is irritated, we look for the source of irritation in the condition of the sewage system of the body, which is the colon.

I have observed again and again that when people have noticed the first indication of a sore throat, the soreness has disappeared almost immediately upon promptly taking a high enema followed by a series of colon irrigations.

I had occasion, many years ago, to take a trip into Mexico which would keep me there for at least two or three weeks. Another doctor accompanied me. The night before leaving, although I did not feel I needed one, I took a high enema. I also took my enema bag and lubricating tube with me in my suitcase. I returned from my trip in perfect health, whereas my doctor friend, who was not as colon-conscious as I was, returned with a dose of amoebic diarrhea.

I am absolutely sure that if my doctor friend had taken some colon irrigations before we went to Mexico, he too would have returned in perfect health. We stayed in the same hotel and we ate all our meals together. Our first luncheon was at the Focolare Restaurant. The head waiter was an Italian whose name was Mr. Sabato. He and I "clicked" instantly when I was able to talk with him in Italian. My friend ordered some meat for his lunch, while my order was for an all-raw vegetable salad served with a dressing which I suggested. When our respective dishes arrived, my friend said my meal looked so good that the next time he would order the same! Now if the cause of his ailment were to afflict every American who visited Mexico, by all such rules I should have been afflicted in the same way he was. But it did not work that way. He developed throat trouble which persisted for three or four weeks.

A number of times I have had students and friends call on me before they were leaving for destinations abroad and, as far as I was able to check, all those who took the necessary colon-cleansing precautions returned after a healthy trip with no ill effects. However, two or three who contacted me on their return told me they were *not* meticulous in the matter of their colons, and they did have some health problems, principally bowel and throat trouble.

So, even if the colon happens to be located two or

three feet away from the throat, with no apparent connection between them, it is an indisputable fact that the relationship exists — obscure as it may seem to be.

The Spine and Its Distribution Network

The **spine**, of course, is man's physical backbone. The **spinal fluid**, however, is something vastly different and as important in its own sphere as the spine is in its physical function.

The spine starts at the base of the skull, continues down in a series of interlocking vertebrae to the solid triangular bone called the sacrum, and ends at the coccyx.

The **cerebrospinal fluid** is a liquid substance only seven to eight one-thousandths heavier than the specific gravity of distilled water. It is the fluid which maintains a constant flow between the brain through the spinal cord, and enables every nerve in the body to bathe its nerve cells in it constantly. The eyeballs are filled with cerebrospinal fluid. In order to better understand the far-reaching influence and effects of this important spinal fluid, one should visualize its main location and means of distribution. Study closely the accompanying illustrations.

In the skull, surrounding the brain, we have, to the touch, the outer bone of the cranium on which the hair grows. Immediately underneath this bone there is an attached membrane known as the dura mater, which has a spider-web-like, fine membrane known as the arachnoid. The arachnoid, in turn, forms the "outer" wall of the canal which encircles the brain and the

THE SPINE

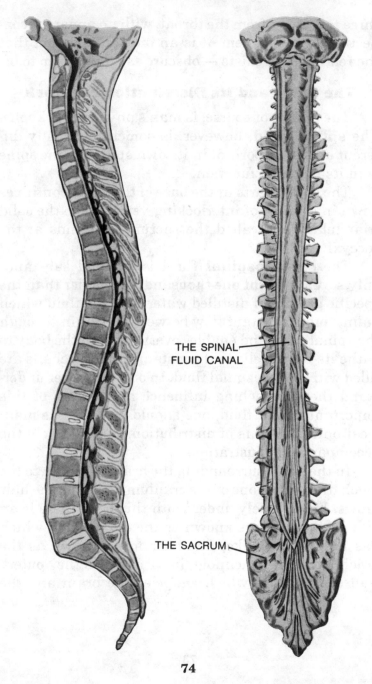

THE SPINAL
FLUID CANAL

THE SACRUM

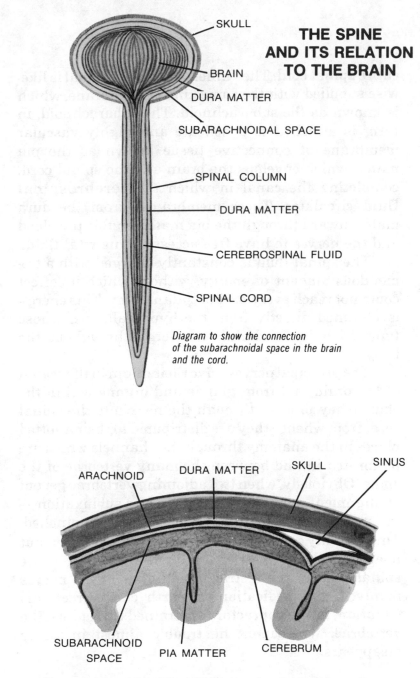

THE SPINE
AND ITS RELATION
TO THE BRAIN

SKULL

BRAIN

DURA MATTER

SUBARACHNOIDAL SPACE

SPINAL COLUMN

DURA MATTER

CEREBROSPINAL FLUID

SPINAL CORD

*Diagram to show the connection
of the subarachnoidal space in the brain
and the cord.*

ARACHNOID

DURA MATTER

SKULL

SINUS

SUBARACHNOID
SPACE

PIA MATTER

CEREBRUM

*Diagram to represent the relations of the meningeal membranes of the cerebrum,
the position of the subarachnoidal space and of the venous sinuses.*

entire spinal cord. The "inner" wall of the canal is likewise supplied with the same kind of membrane, which is known as the subarachnoid. The subarachnoid, in turn, is attached to a delicate and highly vascular membrane of connective tissue known as the pia mater, which envelops the brain and the spinal cord, completing the canal in which the **cerebrospinal fluid** circulates. These membranes, from the dura mater inward through the pia mater, enable the blood and the nerves to have free access to this vital fluid.

The spinal fluid is constantly charged with a tremendous amount of energy, without which its effect could not reach every part of the anatomy. This energy is obtained directly from the hypothalamus, whose function it is to administer energy throughout the body.

The principal nerves have their origin in the region of the brain and from glands and organs within the skull. They proceed through the neck into the spinal cord, from whence they are distributed to their allotted places in the anatomy through the channels which are perforated in and between the many vertebrae of the spine. Obviously, when two adjoining vertebrae get out of alignment — a condition known as a subluxation — the nerves between these vertebrae become pinched. This not only causes pain or discomfort to register, but it also blocks or interferes with the function of the spinal fluid in the restricted activities of the nerves involved. No medication on earth can correct this situation, but chiropractors are trained to re-adjust the vertebrae, whereupon the trouble almost instantly disappears.

What causes such subluxations? In most cases it is stress and tension. Such conditions, in turn, may be caused by many and varied circumstances. One of the most insidious circumstances is the presence of resentment and the hate that so often accompanies it. It is a very rare and unusual person that did not start in childhood to develop resentments. Unless these resentments are completely cleared up so they can be forgiven and forgotten, they may develop into monsters that cause conditions such as arthritis and cancer.

As mentioned previously, one very serious cause of stress, tension and fatigue is the removal of tonsils. In some very mysterious manner tonsils are intimately related to the nerve system of the anatomy and consequently to the spinal fluid.

The value of chiropractic treatments is inestimable because of their intimate relation to both the nerves and the spinal fluid. I know a lady, a senior citizen, who was vivacious, joyful and overflowing with energy while a child. At the age of around eleven or twelve her tonsils were removed. Her early training and upbringing gave her a very proud outlook on life which was of tremendous help in future years. Within a very few months after her tonsillectomy she began gradually to lose both her energy and her innate joyousness, but she was too proud to have people know.

Fortunately she married a chiropractor, whom I have known for many years. I learned that his wife would go through her work and activities like a house afire — as he put it — then suddenly she would have to drop on a couch, utterly exhausted. He taught me a

77

wonderful technique which I want to pass on to my readers. He would have his wife sit at a table and he would get behind her. Beginning at her neck at the base of the skull, he applies considerable pressure on the spine with the knuckles of his first finger on each hand, one knuckle on the right side of the vertebra and the other knuckle on the left side of the vertebra. Keeping the pressure for about ten seconds, he then moves down to the next vertebra, repeating the same procedure for ten seconds on each vertebra until he reaches the sacrum. Then he clenches his fists and starts upward by pressing several vertebrae on each side of the spine with the three knuckles of his middle fingers, just as he did with his forefinger knuckles, until he reaches the neck once again, this time exerting the same pressure for only about six seconds each time. This treatment has a very excellent effect, which may even last a day or two if she has the opportunity to rest as much as she needs to.

Actually, the effect of this pressure on each vertebra is to inhibit any muscles involved in the development of stress or tension. The muscles are thereby relaxed, and this relaxation spreads throughout the entire body. This treatment has also been very effective when a person has trouble going to sleep.

The spinal fluid is replete with trace elements in greater volume and variety than any other organ in the body. These elements are distributed throughout the body by means of the blood and nerves, which collect these trace elements from the spinal fluid. To appreciate the importance and value of these trace elements you must realize, for example, that many of them are so evanescent that only about 10 or 15 milligrams (a fraction of an ounce of some of them) could be extracted from 2,000 pounds — one ton — of alfalfa, which is one of our richest sources of trace elements.

Excessive fermentation and putrefaction are the spinal fluid's worst enemies. To cause **anything** to impair the effectiveness of this vital fluid would almost be analogous to building-up premature senility and possibly, a painful demise.

Do not, for one moment, underestimate the vigor with which I advocate the need to cleanse the colon by means of colon irrigations. The life they save may well be **yours**.

What was that you asked me? Do I take colon irrigations? I most certainly **do**! In fact, I have just this past week concluded my series of six irrigations in three weeks — two a week.

THE BRONCHIALS AND THE LUNGS

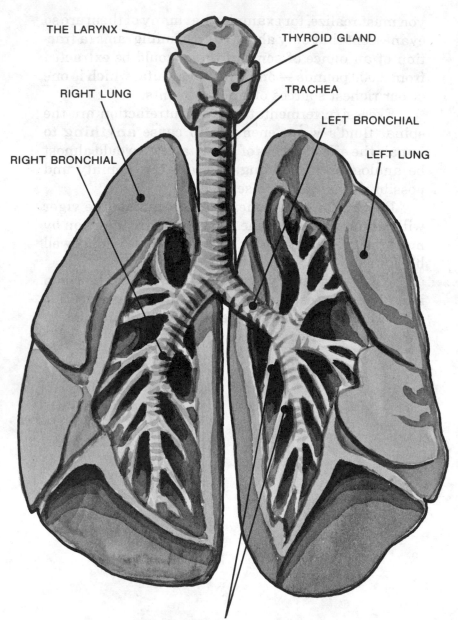

THE LARYNX

THYROID GLAND

RIGHT LUNG

TRACHEA

LEFT BRONCHIAL

RIGHT BRONCHIAL

LEFT LUNG

DORSAL BRONCHIAL BRANCHES

Chapter 6.
The Chest —
Your Body's Vitality Center

The Trachea

The **trachea**, or windpipe, extends from the larynx to the bronchial tubes. It lies against the front surface of the esophagus, is flanked on its sides by the arteries, veins and nerves of the neck, and is positioned behind the thymus gland. It is in close relationship to the large blood vessels entering and leaving the heart.

The trachea is larger in the male than in the female. In the child it is smaller, more deeply placed and more movable than in the adult.

In the neck, the trachea lies in relation to the two lobes of the thyroid gland. Goiter is likely to affect the breathing apparatus because of the constriction which takes place from the swelling in the neck.

The trachea is greatly affected by the accumulation of mucus in the sinuses and, in fact, by the presence of excessive amounts of phlegm and mucus in the throat.

The larynx is part and parcel of the respiratory system and of the trachea, and is what we would call the voice box. It is the organ by means of which we are able to speak, sing, shout, and loudly praise the Lord for giving us such a miraculous instrument with which to express ourselves vocally.

The larynx is situated between the trachea and the base of the tongue. It consists of a number of cartilages or grist-like tissues such as the thyroid cartilage, the epiglottis cartilage, the cricoid cartilage and three other pairs. They are lined by a mucous membrane and are moved or operated by the muscles of the larynx. The mucous membrane forms into two folds which constitute the vocal bands, the upper being the false, and the lower the true vocal band. The changes in the pitch of the voice are provided by the approximation or separation of these bands. The space between the vocal bands is called the glottis. In birds the vocal cord is called the syrinx, or lower larynx, and is located at the division of the branches of the trachea.

The larynx is continuous with the trachea at its lower end and opens above in the pharynx. This opening is reduced to a T-shaped interval during the act of swallowing by the mechanism or operation of the epiglottis. The larynx is the valve in the trachea which prevents liquids and solids from entering the air passage in the lungs. Its position is particularly evident in men, as it is known as the **Adam's apple** or laryngeal prominence.

When the body — and the colon in particular — is overloaded with waste matter in a state of fermentation and putrefaction, the larynx is easily susceptible to inflammation, which may be acute or chronic, from catarrh, from pus, or it can be due to diphtheria, tuberculosis or syphilis. All of these conditions have responded in a satisfactory manner to the application of colon irrigations.

Consider the handicap of not being able to speak! A series of colon irrigations, from long past experience, has enabled so very many people of all ages to correct many disturbances. It is well worth remembering whenever any physical affliction overtakes us to take a series of cleansings; however, prevention is always the best policy, particularly when it concerns the matter of health.

The Esophagus

The **esophagus**, or gullet, is a muscular canal about nine inches in length, extending from the pharynx to the stomach. It passes down the neck between the trachea and the spinal column. Passing behind the left branch of the bronchial tubes, it pierces the diaphragm slightly to the left of its middle line and then joins the heart end of the stomach.

A gradual change takes place in the function of the esophagus as the voluntary muscular activity, of which we are conscious, changes to the involuntary muscle activity and forms the process of propulsion of food from the mouth to the stomach.

The chemical action to prepare our food for digestion starts in the mouth when we masticate our food, converting it into a heterogenous mass, or bolus. This is saturated with the secretion of our combined parotid, submaxillary, sublingual and mucous glands of the mouth, ordinarily known as saliva. The function of the saliva is to moisten the food, to lubricate the bolus, to dissolve certain substances, to help deglutition (the process of swallowing the food), and generally to help digestion. This whole process takes place in the mouth, so that the esophagus has nothing more to do than to propel the bolus from the mouth to the stomach.

Naturally, when the body is afflicted with vast quantities of mucus within the area of the head, some of the mucus is bound to filter through the esophagus. As this mucus is a natural magnet for pathogenic germs and bacteria, there is the danger of these parasites slipping into the esophagus within the bolus. As the digestive system has no selective ability or powers, it is a simple matter for them to get into the stomach and small intestine where they can really play havoc.

Obviously, thorough cleanliness is the price of health, and we have found that colon irrigations at all stages of the condition of our systems are an invaluable means to give us assurance that the beneficial germs and bacteria will take care of whatever situation may arise.

By living naturally and eating the foods which regenerate the cells and tissues of the body, keeping our mind on a high plane of consciousness, we can help every organ in the body, including the esophagus, to work for us faithfully for a longer and healthier life.

Vulgarity, coarseness, and ribaldry are all indicative of a morbid state of consciousness, of an immoral state of mind. Such a manner of living is very damaging to the body functions and is a definite degenerating factor, detrimental and injurious to the brain cells. The study of criminals has proven that this deleterious state of mind and body has been the primary contributing factor in leading the individual into a life of crime.

To avoid this distressing state of affairs from afflicting the family, discipline and proper training of children is essential. As the child grows he is forming the habits which will dominate his life as an adult.

Bronchials and the Lungs

The trachea, the **bronchials** and the **lungs** are a continuous channel through which the air that we breathe must pass in order that the blood stream can collect the oxygen and the nitrogen which the body requires to keep us alive.

The bronchials, which are an extension of the trachea, divert the air through the entire area of the right and left lobes of the lungs. This action prevents excessive accumulation of air in any one spot, to the harm or detriment of that particular spot, or elsewhere.

The bronchials are lined with a cellular tissue consisting of layers of cells, the hair-like fingers of which lead upwards towards the throat to carry mucus and other extraneous material away from the lungs into the pharynx for elimination. This lining is composed of lymphatic vessels, nerves and small blood vessels. There is an under-lining, known as the submucosa, which contains larger blood vessels and glands known as trachea glands, whose ducts open through the mucous lining to the open surface of the first lining.

For a very definite protective purpose, the diameter of the right bronchus was created larger than that of the left one. If an object that has no business getting into the lungs should enter the windpipe, it will automatically go through the right bronchus without affecting the lung connected with the left bronchus. What foresight!

If you could see a cross-section of your body at about the level of the breast bone, in the center you would see the area of the heart, with the sternum or breast bone in front and the spinal bones in the back. On each side you would see the right and the left lobes of the lungs, with the root of the lungs on the level of a vertebra's inner surface.

Completely surrounding the lungs is a sack-like tissue known as the pleura, which consists of a canal known as the pleural cavity, which is enclosed on the lung side of the canal by a tissue known as the visceral pleura, and on the other side of the canal by a similar tissue known as the parietal (or costal) pleura. When the health condition of the body is below par, one may be sitting in a draft and shortly feel a sharp pain as if someone had pushed a knife into your ribs. A doctor would tell you that you have contracted **pleurisy**.

The pleura is an elastic structure. It is on this account that, when we do get bitten by such an agonizing pain, the sharp thrusts are the result of the expansion and contraction of the lung within the pleura which squeezes the sensitive fluid in the pleural cavity. Prolonged affliction of the pleura causes inflammation which becomes progressively afflicting.

Because the liver lies just below the root of the right lung, it has a tendency to push the lung upward. This makes the right lung shorter and broader than the left lung, but in actual volume it is larger. The left lung, although longer, has less volume-capacity than the right lung because the heart occupies a considerable portion of the left thorax.

Through the act of breathing, the lungs are able to give the blood a constant supply of oxygen, without which we could not stay alive more than a few minutes. The lungs also collect the nitrogen from the air we breathe, and this nitrogen is used to replenish the amino acids composing the protein in the system.

The lungs are of a light, porous, spongy texture which floats in water. They are connected with the bronchials by a great many branches of bronchi which spread throughout the several lobes of the lungs, becoming progressively smaller until they measure only about one millimeter in diameter. At this stage they are called bronchioles.

The lungs are replete with myriads of tiny sacs like microscopic bunches of grapes, called alveoli, which actually deposit the air we breathe into the blood vessels which abound in the area and collect from that same blood, the carbon dioxide which must be removed from the system with every expulsion of our breath. In this manner our breathing constitutes a constant in-breathing of air and out-breathing of carbon dioxide. Notwithstanding the multiplicity of alveoli in the lungs, any air pollution that we breathe into our lungs has its definite harmful effect on the condition of our health.

The atmosphere of the city, which is replete with carbon monoxide (the deadly exhaust from internal combustion engines), gasoline, kerosene and similar hydrocarbon products, is responsible for a great many respiratory ailments and ailments resulting in carbon monoxide pollution of the blood. This is, without question, one of the many reasons why intelligent people who are able to do so have been moving to the open country in recent years.

Tobacco smoke is particularly deadly, as indicated by autopsies of cadavers of people who smoked tobacco most of their lives. The alveoli were destroyed in dangerously vast numbers, leaving the color of the lung black as coal.

While your life is in your blood, the air you breathe is a contributing factor in determining the length of your life span and the state of your later years of life, whether these will be healthy and happy — or end in a decrepit senility.

The condition of the entire breathing apparatus, from the mouth and the nostrils through the trachea, the bronchials, and through your lungs, depends on the cleanliness of the colon as well as the lungs. There is no escaping this phase of the care of the body. Fermentation and putrefaction in the colon have their effect on the health of every part of the anatomy and, consequently, on the body as a whole. We have found through the years that every person coming to our attention with bronchial and other breathing problems, who cleansed their body by means of a series of colon irrigations, found relief from their affliction and frequently discovered the loss of other ailments which had been bothering them.

The Thyroid Gland

The **thyroid gland** is located at the front and sides of the neck and consists of the right and left lobes which are connected across the middle by a narrow strip called the isthmus. The thyroid is slightly heavier in the female than in the male and becomes somewhat enlarged during menstruation and pregnancy.

There is very close communication between the lymph vessels and the blood vessels in the capsule of the thyroid gland. The nerves are a mass of tissue derivating from the sympathetic nerve system of the neck. The thyroid is a gland of internal secretion, which means that it has no ducts through which secretions can escape, except directly into the lymph stream and into the blood vessels. When the thyroid is called upon to supply these secretions to the system, the vesicles in which they are generated break open, and the secretion is collected by the lymph stream and carried where called for. These secretions are thyroid hormones which the body needs not only for purposes of metabolism, but also for growth and development.

Iodine is one of the most important nutritional requirements of the thyroid gland. Did I say iodine is **one** of the most important? Iodine is by far **the most** essential trace element needed by the thyroid gland in particular, and by the entire body in general. The importance of iodine was never brought home to my consciousness more than when I happened to be giving some lectures in Charleston, West Virginia. I had occasion to call on a doctor in Clendenin, a small town of some 1,200 or 1,400 inhabitants. He showed me two bot-

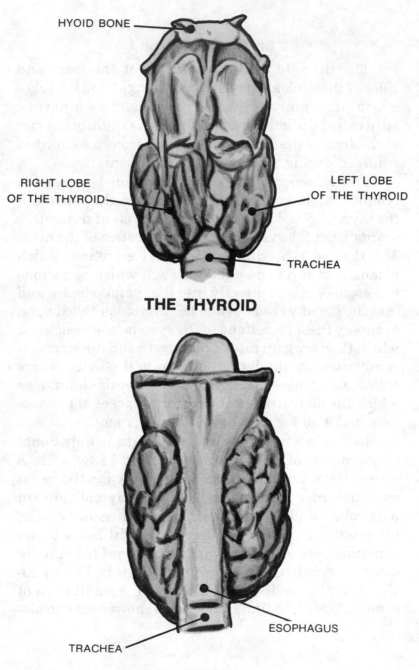

HYOID BONE

RIGHT LOBE
OF THE THYROID

LEFT LOBE
OF THE THYROID

TRACHEA

THE THYROID

ESOPHAGUS

TRACHEA

tles containing salt, one from a salt mine nearby, the other pure white table salt. He told me that when his father, who also was a doctor, first came there goiter was something unkown. At that time, pure white table salt was making its appearance in the grocery stores, and within a few years a high percentage of goiters had made their appearance in alarming numbers. The reason? Natives had always used the salt just as it came from the local mines. This local salt contained a percentage of iodine; however, the pure white table salt contained none! When this became known, the table salt made a quick exit from that area, and by the use of the mined salt most of the goiters diminished and many disappeared.

The ability of the thyroid to utilize iodine is related to the extent that the cleansing of the colon is maintained. This is particularly noticeable when an incipient goiter makes its appearance. A series of colon irrigations have considerably speeded utilization of organic iodine by the thyroid, the vanishing of the incipient goiter, and recovery of mental alertness.

Iodine is the basic ingredient of the hormone thyroxin. When the thyroid for any reason is unable to generate sufficient thyroxin, the skin attains a peculiar graying tint and bloats or thickens, the hair becomes dry and brittle, the body weight increases, and, worst of all, there is a loss of vigor and mentality. This condition is similar to that experienced after a tonsillectomy, indicating the close relationship between the thyroid and the tonsils, which are both seriously influenced by the condition of the colon.

This iodine deficiency must be given serious consideration by folks living in areas which have been found to be afflicted with considerable incidences of goiter, as in parts of Michigan, Minnesota and Wisconsin, and equally prevalent in the states of Washington, Oregon and the mountain regions of Colorado. In these areas it is particularly important to use colon irrigations several times during the year, and in order to remedy the iodine deficiency some organic iodine should be part of the daily diet (dulse and granulated kelp).

The average adult requirement of iodine is mighty small — only about one quarter of a milligram is figured as the minimum daily need. Half a level teaspoon of powdered or granulated kelp is ample. This can be mixed with any kind of food, the best being raw salads and raw vegetable juices.

Here is where the benefit of living on your own little farm in the country comes in. If you put 20 to 40 pounds of potassium iodide per acre in your soil, you will be able to have a sufficient supply of iodine with everything you eat that is grown in that soil. If you keep poultry and other livestock, you could feed them potassium iodide with benefit both to them and to you. In fact, many farmers have found that in feeding potassium iodide to their poultry, the eggs contained as much as 400% more iodine than eggs from poultry without this additive. The same is true of milk from goats and cows fed potassium iodide.

My greatest objection to iodized salt is the fact that, apart from the benefit which may be derived from the iodine, its danger has not been eliminated because it has been heated to tremendous temperatures to make it pour.

The importance of water balance in the body must not be overlooked, as the thyroid is intimately involved in this process. The human body is composed of between 75% and 80% distilled water. If insufficient water fails to furnish the necessary humidity to the waste matter in the colon, constipation develops, as well as hard stools which are painful and difficult to excrete. Thus, equal attention must be given both to the thyroid and the colon.

The body's metabolism is dependent on the thyroid hormone thyroxin for its proper function; in these areas both the thyroid and the colon are very intimately involved.

The thyroid gland is controlled by the pituitary gland, which we have already discussed in a preceding chapter. This pituitary control, in turn, is administered by the hypothalamus in the mid-brain. It does not take any great stretch of the imagination to realize what a wonderful, miraculous organ our Eternal Creator conceived. He created it, as He did everything else, **with perfection**. It is man in his free will, with which he was endowed, who has degraded his body by heeding his appetite instead of nourishing his body with the **natural**, unspoiled, unprocessed food intended for nourishment, replenishment and regeneration.

The Thymus Gland

The **thymus gland** is quite large in infants and

THE THYMUS

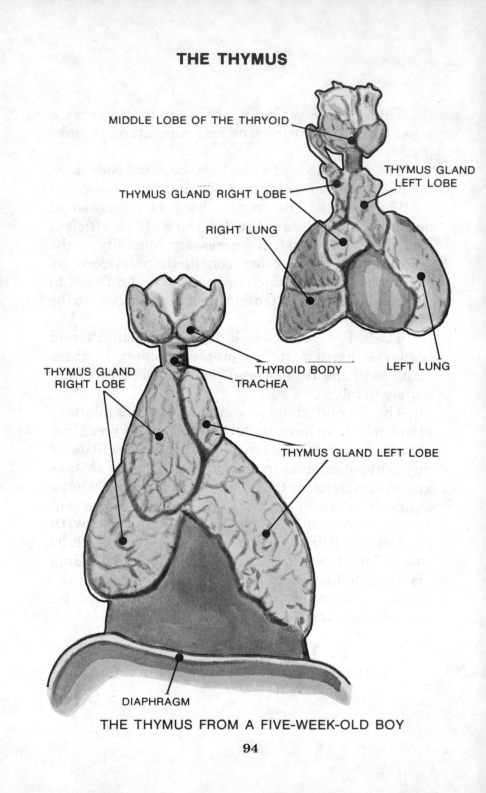

MIDDLE LOBE OF THE THRYOID

THYMUS GLAND LEFT LOBE

THYMUS GLAND RIGHT LOBE

RIGHT LUNG

LEFT LUNG

THYMUS GLAND RIGHT LOBE

THYROID BODY

TRACHEA

THYMUS GLAND LEFT LOBE

DIAPHRAGM

THE THYMUS FROM A FIVE-WEEK-OLD BOY

94

children, but after puberty it gradually shrinks. A boy only five-weeks-old will have a very large thymus. The thymus of an adult person would be only a fraction of the size of a child's.

In the past this gland was considered to have run its course and outlived its usefulness at puberty. It is now known that the thymus has a very close relationship with the reproductive organs throughout life; this relationship begins at birth and continues on a definite course during the development of the reproductive system. During the period of adolescence, the gland becomes more or less nervously agitated and responds closely to the tonsils. Consequently, when the tonsils are removed, the agitation of the thymus causes the reproductive system to undergo serious psychological changes closely akin to what happens to a man who is castrated. We have seen, in our preceding chapter on tonsils, how far-reaching the changes can be in both men and women. The thymus has, so to speak, its own hand in that change.

The gradual loss of maximum sex productivity and excitement can be better understood when considering the progressive loss in the weight of the thymus. At birth its weight is about 15 grams; upon reaching puberty the weight has increased to 35 grams; at the age of 25 it has decreased to 25 grams; at the age of 60 it weighs about 15 grams, while at 70 it gets down to about 6 grams. To me, this steady decrease from puberty to old age portrays a most telling and interesting story of what everybody has noticed. The more frequently a man during his prime years wastes the vital forces, the more rapid is the loss in weight of the thymus. Consequently, this is a decisive factor in premature senility and a shorter life span.

The thymus is equipped with glands of internal secretion which are related to those of the reproductive organs. The blood supply to the thymus is derived from the internal mammary glands in the breast and from the thyroid. The thyroid is a particularly important gland in our anatomical economy. A disturbance of the thymus can be reflected in, or from, any of the reproductive organs, the mammary glands or the thyroid. Likewise, such a disturbance could be related to, or from, this particular spot on the cecum of the ascending colon.

During adolescence the outside coating of the thymus gland begins to acquire fatty tissues until, during the middle twenties, a considerable coating of fat has accumulated. Apparently the purpose of this fat is for the production of antibodies and immunizing material, which are passed into the lymph stream by the many lymph glands present in the thymus. These antibodies are antagonistic to the harmful action of bacteria, germs and pathogenic microorganisms. The antibodies are characteristic constituents of the blood and fluids of the body. In other words, the thymus becomes a manufacturing plant for the production of antitoxins, counter-poisons and antidotes which counteract toxins throughout the system. These antitoxins fight disease, as well as build up immunity. This procedure works splendidly, as long as the body, and the colon in particular, is in a perfectly healthy condition.

When the colon is neglected and the lymph stream becomes overloaded with waste matter which it is unable to dispose of, then the lymph fluid begins to store up waste matter in the lymph glands throughout the system, a purpose for which these lymph glands were created. When these lymph glands are filled to the limit of their capacity, trouble develops usually in the form of lumps in a few or in many parts of the body. One can appreciate the cooperation which exists between the colon and the lymph stream.

As we have already observed, the thymus is intimately related to the mammary glands in the breast. It is understandable, therefore, that these sensitive mammary glands would be an easy target for the formation of lumps, which is what frequently happens. Unfortunately, this condition has developed the all too frequent practice of removing the breast by means of surgery, on the assumption that the lump was malignant.

During the past decade quite a number of ladies, usually aged from mid-30's and older, asked for counsel and advice because breast removal had been recommended. Most of them heeded our opinion and promptly had a series of colon irrigations which cleared up the lumps usually in a matter of days!

One particularly interesting case was a lady I did not know, who telephoned me from New York to tell me she had just run out of the hospital where she had gone for observation to determine the cause and condition of lumps all over her body. The night before, while in bed in the hospital, she became curious to see what her card in the rack at the foot of the bed had to say about her condition. She was shocked to read that she was due to go to the operating room the next morning for an exploratory investigation for cancer. She promptly jumped out of bed, dressed, and rushed home. I told her it would be useless for her to come all the way to Arizona when she could perfectly well be taken care of in New York. I told her that if I were so afflicted I would, without delay, take a series of colon irrigations on consecutive days for about three weeks. She said that was exactly what she would do. I asked her to let me hear from her in the next three or four weeks and let me know how she was. She telephoned me a month later to tell me that every single lump had disappeared from her body, and she felt such wonderful energy and vitality that she hardly knew what to do with herself. Of course, I should add that she drank several pints of fresh raw vegetable juices and followed our program as closely as she could every day during that month, and she intended to continue to do so. Exciting, is it not?

The lumps in this lady's case were the result of failing to keep the colon clean. The condition of the colon was caused by ingestion of incompatible foods, foods cooked in oil and grease, and by drinking beverages which contributed to the disturbance of the digestive system. Living in New York, she all too frequently ate in restaurants where she was not able to control the quality of the food, nor the manner in which it was handled and cooked. It took the scare of a cancer operation to convert her into eating natural foods.

Besides the relationship which the thymus gland

has with the thyroid and the mammary glands, it also has some direct or indirect relationship with both the adrenal glands and the solar plexus. All these centers are involved in both emotional and sexual feelings.

A disturbance in this particular area of the colon frequently results from excessive mucus production as a result of eating and drinking mucous-forming foods. Of these, cow's milk is the worst offender. I have noticed that children brought up drinking quantities of cow's milk are by far more readily disturbed emotionally than children who were breast-fed to at least 18 months and who drank fresh raw goat's milk and fresh raw vegetable juices. These latter children were invariably more emotionally stable and better disciplined.

As for adults, when the nature of the ingested food consists of an undue proportion of meats, fried and grease-cooked foods, and the colon is not clean, there is the tendency to find a sexual over-stimulation and the concomitant perversions associated therewith.

Never underestimate the value of your thymus gland. Almighty God had many good reasons for placing it right where it is. It is your responsibility, therefore, to watch your food and keep your colon washed and healthy while you still have it.

The Heart

We are now on our way across the transverse colon (please refer to the *Colon Therapy Chart* for location), and we have arrived at the area marked **heart**. The heart is purely and simply an automatic organ. The automaticity of the beat of the heart results from

THE HEART

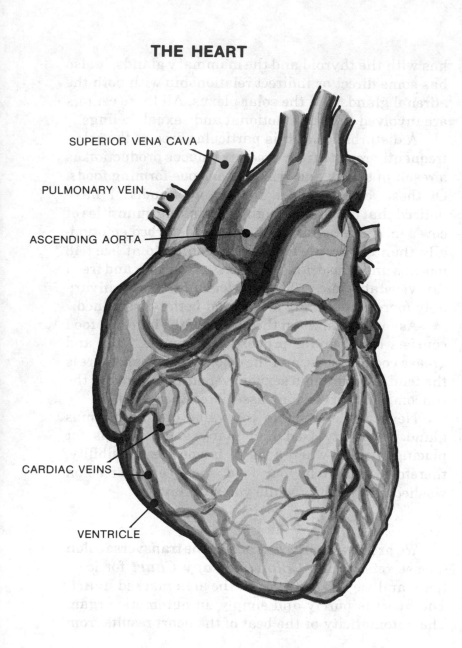

SUPERIOR VENA CAVA

PULMONARY VEIN

ASCENDING AORTA

CARDIAC VEINS

VENTRICLE

the function of both the muscles and the nerves with which the heart is equipped; however, these alone do not contain the activating force which keeps the normal, healthy heart striking some 100,000 beats each day for 50, 75, 100 years and more. Yet this miraculous pump is just about the size of a man's fist.

The entire body contains only about five quarts of blood. This is its entire supply of blood, and a healthy body does not add any more to it throughout its entire life. Nevertheless, during each 24-hour period, day after day, year in and year out, this tiny pump, the heart, pumps between 10,000 and 11,000 quarts of blood throughout the body from head to foot. Just think, during a mere 50 years the heart will have pumped some **45 million gallons of blood through your system**. Miraculous? No human contrivance could begin to equal that performance. Yet Almighty God created man in His image and contrived this degree of perfection. For whose benefit was this? For your benefit and for mine.

Wherein lies the secret of such constant, timely and efficient service? It lies right in your mid-brain, in a mass of nerves known as the hypothalamus. As you have learned in the chapter on the hypothalamus, this organ is the transformer which lowers the cosmic energy vibrations of the universe from untold millions of volts down to the degree of energy-voltage which the individual needs from moment to moment. Thus, the hypothalamus administers the perpetual motion of cosmic energy by some computerizing means which we have not yet discovered, caring for the needs of the glands, organs and parts of the body.

One of the prerequisites of the normal activity of the heart is the constant state of cleanliness of the colon. If there is an excessive accumulation of waste matter fermenting and putrefying in the colon, the results will affect the heart.

Some years ago, I had a telephone call about 11 o'clock one night from a lady in Kansas. I did not know her, but I did remember that she had bought one of my *Foot Relaxation Charts*. She told me her father was having a heart attack and she did not want to call a medical doctor.

I said to her, "You have my *Foot Relaxation Chart*, if I remember rightly?"

"Yes," she said. "I have it framed right in my room."

I said to her, "You see where the sole of the foot..."

She interrupted me with the emphatic remark, "But my father is having a **heart** attack. His feet are all right!"

I continued, "You see where the picture of the heart is on the sole of the foot? If I were you I would take his shoes off and take his foot in both my hands and press with my finger tips on the area of the picture of the heart, with as much pressure as I could use, and keep it up for about 15 minutes."

She telephoned me again two days later to tell me she did this and in a few minutes her father started belching and passing foul-smelling gas in volumes from his bowels. He then slept soundly till nine o'clock the next morning and was back in his office that day.

Concentrated starchy foods can cause a great deal of trouble in the colon and can also be dangerous for the heart. The digestion of such starches in excessive quantities causes the creation of abnormal amounts of carbon which becomes carbonic acid gas. To avoid this danger we need to reduce our consumption of starches to a minimum or, better still, avoid them.

Let me clarify this principle of the automatic function of the heart. The rhythmical contractions of the heart must essentially be a phenomenon originating outside of, and apart from, the cells and tissues of the heart, which are purely physical matter. There is no physical matter which can exercise any activity 24 hours a day for 80, 90 or more than 100 years without needing to be repaired over and over again. This does not take place in the heart. Therefore, it is obvious that the automatic function of the heart comes from some extraneous, ephemeral source. That source is unquestionably superhuman. Cosmic energy **is** superhuman, and so are the cosmic energy vibrations emanating from the hypothalamus, transmitted there to the heart by some mysterious computerized system. This would account for the fact that the heart of a healthy vigorous man of 80, 90 and even 100 years of age has not stopped its heartbeat for one single instant. Physiologists have been calling this quasi-perpetual motion an "inward stimulus," and so it is, emanating from the universe. Almighty God certainly accomplished a perfect masterpiece when he created man's heart.

The heart is very definitely affected by impurities in the blood — and by fermentation and putrefaction of waste matter anywhere in the system — because these impurities are collected by both the blood and the lymph. The blood and the lymph fluid passes through the heart constantly. Gases from the colon can readily pass into any part of the body by the process of gas-osmosis. Obviously when a pocket of gas forms any-where in the heart area it is very likely to cause trouble, whether the gas is inside the transverse colon or in the area of the diaphragm. At the beginning of the dissertation in this chapter, I have given a graphic example of how a heart attack can take place under such conditions, and how by relaxing the muscles in the area involved the trouble has been dissipated and the heart attack vanished.

There are three particular mineral elements which the heart needs, essential only in very small amounts — a mere fraction of one percent. These are potassium, sodium and calcium. The potassium and the sodium promote a state of relaxation in the muscles, while the calcium promotes a state of contraction. These ele-ments are supplied by the food we eat. When the food is raw, these elements are in the form of organic minerals which are readily assimilated for constructive pur-poses by the body. When these elements are obtained from cooked or fried food, they are inorganic and much of their energy and value is lost. Fortunately, the body is equipped with a vast degree of tolerance and can util-ize such inorganic elements, but it does so at the expense of much waste of energy in the processes of digestion. Cooked and fried foods create far more fer-mentation and putrefaction than do the live, organic foods.

The blood is the life of the body, while the heart is

the motor which keeps that life in circulation. The regular function and activity of the heart is essential for our survival. Once we become thoroughly conscious of this, we will do everything in our power to keep the body in tip-top shape — inside and out. However, keeping the body perserved within is by far more important because we cannot know if anything is wrong until an affliction, ailment or sickness suddenly warns us of the fact. In order to attain this tip-top shape one should concentrate on the colon — experience has taught me there is nothing more important than this.

There is no organ in the body which can be tampered with or removed without some unpredictable damage or danger occurring in the future. If at all possible, it is the better part of wisdom never to part with any organ, gland, or necessary part of the anatomy. Always remember that while Almighty God made your body perfect in the very beginning, He has also supplied us with the manner and means whereby we can remedy whatever transgressions to which we have subjected our body.

The Diaphragm

We do not often hear the word **diaphragm** spoken in connection with our anatomy. It is usually referred to as the midriff. Actually, the diaphragm is the partition which separates the cavity of the chest from that of the abdomen. It is attached to the lumbar vertebrae in the back, and to the sixth or seventh ribs and their cartilages. When a person breathes the diaphragm contracts, flattens and increases the capacity of the thorax.

The diaphragm is a very important muscular structure involved in breathing, in defecation, in the bodily activity during childbirth, and in other processes. When one has hiccups the diaphragm contracts in spasms. The muscles in the back of the diaphragm extend all the way from the sacrum, at the bottom of the spinal column, to the skull, thus being subject to troubles which may afflict the spine.

The diaphragm muscles in the thoracic area causes elevation and depression of the ribs when breathing. There is a very effective exercise which I indulge in nearly every time I take a walk. It consists of blowing through the teeth to the sound of "SHOO-SHOO-Shoo-shoo-shoo," repeated over and over again. Just try it, place your hand on your diaphragm, go "SHOO-SHOO-Shoo-shoo-shoo," and you will feel the diaphragm drawing inward. This means that you are forcing the stale air and carbon dioxide out of the lower part of your lungs and automatically, as if by a vacuum, you unconsciously draw into your lower lung a supply of fresh air. When I take my mile walk I always practice this, the ground seems to just slide past me, and I return feeling refreshed. A little practice will reveal the inward significance of this exercise. It was the late Dr. Thomas Gaines that taught me this about 40 years ago. I have climbed some of the mountains around here, such as Squaw Peak, without a flutter of a heartbeat or puffing, unlike most of the people with which I have walked.

The activities in which the diaphragm is involved are far too numerous to be enumerated here. Suffice it to say that it is actually one of the most important parts of the anatomy, and is very much dependent on the condition of the colon. If we consider the problem of defecation alone, we can understand why it is necessary to keep the colon clean in order to avoid complications in the midriff when being obliged to use muscular force in the region of the rectum when defecation is difficult. Any complication which afflicts the diaphragm can involve breathing, affect the action of the heart, interfere with the digestion and assimilation of food, and cause pressure on the solar plexus, involving the emotions.

It is always wise, useful and foresighted to have a series of colon irrigations at least once every year throughout life. It pays — as nothing can compensate for preventing premature senility or, for that matter, a state of senility at any age.

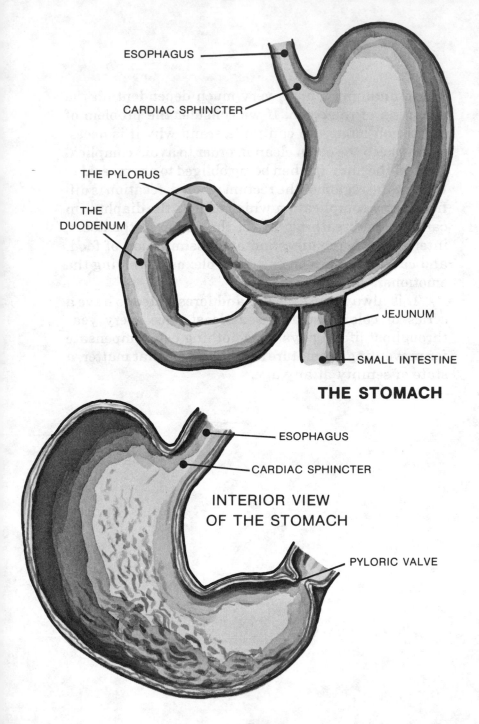

ESOPHAGUS

CARDIAC SPHINCTER

THE PYLORUS

THE
DUODENUM

JEJUNUM

SMALL INTESTINE

THE STOMACH

ESOPHAGUS

CARDIAC SPHINCTER

INTERIOR VIEW
OF THE STOMACH

PYLORIC VALVE

Chapter 7.
The Processing Center
The Stomach

Your **stomach** is either your friend or your enemy, depending on what you put into it.

As long as you are up and around no one can put anything in your stomach except you. What goes into your stomach determines what will eventually be in your colon; you cannot escape this fact. To say "you are what you eat" is a cliche' with much truth in it. The cells and tissues in your body are your servants and are dependent on **you** for their nourishment. They are constantly and faithfully at work for you, day and night, for as many years as you give them the opportunity to regenerate themselves with life by means of the food you eat.

To understand the operation of the stomach we should study the method by which the food we put in our mouth reaches the stomach. As you will have noticed in studying the larynx, it is the valve which shuts off the windpipe when we put something in our mouth which is intended for the stomach. Overlaying the two lips of the larynx is a membrane called the glottis, and over the glottis there is an additional membrane called the epiglottis, which insures the closing of the windpipe allowing the impulsion of food, or any substance, towards the esophagus for delivery into the stomach. In this manner the human body has taken the necessary precautions to prevent our choking to death every time we swallow something. The opening and closing of the glottis is as instantaneous as it is complex, because not a second elapses between the closing of the glottis and the entrance of the food into the esophagus on its way to the stomach. The speed of the passage of the food through the esophagus depends upon its consistency. When the food ingested is very soft or liquid it reaches the entrance to the stomach in about one-tenth of a second by the force of the initial act of swallowing. When the food is solid or semi-solid it is forced down towards the stomach by the action of the peristaltic muscles of the esophagus, usually taking several seconds to reach the stomach.

At the upper end of the stomach there is a sphincter or ring-like muscle which can contract or close the opening into the stomach. This is called the cardiac sphincter and it is controlled both by the vagus nerve, which functions in digestive activities, and the ganglion, known as the semilunar ganglion, which is a group of nerves having their root in the solar plexus. These are closely influenced by the adrenal glands.

The nerve roots in the solar plexus should weave a picture in your mind. The solar plexus is the first organ in the body to "tighten up" whenever there is the slightest mental or emotional disturbance taking place in the individual. Consequently, any such disturbance is bound to affect the digestion at its very beginning. It usually takes only half as long for food to reach the bottom of the stomach as it did to reach the cardiac sphincter from the mouth. The constrictive effect of negative emotions on the solar plexus can be transmitted to the cardiac sphincter, resulting in any of the digestive disturbances.

This relationship between the solar plexus, the adrenal glands, and the cardiac sphincter also has much influence on the period of digestion. Some people can gulp down their food with no apparent harmful results, but such a practice throws the digestive glands, sphincter, and activities out of their normal rhythm, eventually causing a prolapsed stomach, indigestion, and even ulcers in the digestive organs. A slow eater who thoroughly insalivates the food in the mouth assists the digestive processes considerably, provided of course that the food eaten is of a compatible combination.

The manner in which the food is prepared by mastication and insalivation has considerable influence in the processes of digestion and in the ultimate emission of the fiber and other non-digestible material from the small intestine into the cecum pouch of the ascending colon. The finer the mastication, the easier is the work of the digestive glands and the liver.

Once the food gets into the stomach it is entirely cut off from any activity or passage through any part of the digestive system, except during the seconds when the pyloric valve opens to let a minimal amount of the liquefied bolus pass through at regular intervals. This allows the various gastric juices in the stomach to work on the specific type of mineral-chemical elements of which the food eaten was composed. There is a definite orderliness in the movement of the stomach, especially in the separation and ejection of the more liquid parts of the bolus from the more solid.

The dome or fundus of the stomach is not, as many suppose, to cushion air which is expelled when burping. It has been put there for the stomach to use as a storage place for retaining the bulk of food while the activity of the pylorus macerates the bolus and passes it out into the duodenum from time to time. The movement of the bolus starts within a few minutes after it has entered the stomach.

The stomach is flat and in a state of collapse until food is eaten. Then each subsequent mouthful takes its turn in being processed by the gastric juices between the cardiac sphincter and the pylorus. Carbohydrate foods pass from the stomach soon after ingestion and require only about half the time required by proteins for complete gastric processing. Fats, however, when eaten alone remain in the stomach a long time, but when combined with other foods their passage through the pylorus is considerably delayed. Fats are digested by the heat of the body and this heat is regulated by the nerves which are involved in the digestive processes of the stomach.

When a carbohydrate food is eaten before the ingestion of a protein food, the carbohydrate, having the advantage of a priority position, will pass through the pylorus and enter the duodenum promptly, while the protein is delayed for its gastric processing. If, on the other hand, the protein is eaten before the carbohydrate, the passage of the carbohydrate out of the stomach will be retarded. When carbohydrate and protein foods of a concentrated nature are eaten together, the bolus of such a combination is treated first by the protein enzymes in the upper part of the stomach, and the carbohydrate food is thereby "contaminated." When, at its allotted time, the bolus reaches the middle part of the stomach, further acidulation by hydrochloric acid takes place. The result of this delay causes the carbohydrate food to remain in the stomach longer than necessary for its own enzyme processing; this is likely to result in its eventual fermentation along its way towards absorption and elimination. This condition has a serious bearing on a person's elimination problems.

In our present state of civilization, man either requires money with which to buy his food or depends on welfare and becomes a ward of the community. Unfortunately, man is the victim of his appetites. He eats whatever he wants and at any time he chooses. He is influenced by the environment in which he was born and also by the customs and habits of society. He may consequently adopt the same eating habits of those in his environment which, in the final analysis, may turn out to be poison for him.

The colon is the best indicator of a person's habits and of the condition of his body, whether the body is healthy or not. To have a clean colon is the best health insurance we can have. There is no better way that we have found for attaining and maintaining a clean, healthy colon than by means of colon irrigations and eating the right food.

If we were able to live out in the country and grow

our own food organically, we should have no constipation or elimination trouble. After all, farm life may be a life of hard work, but nothing in life is worth having that we do not work for. Farm life could give us all the nutritious foods we need without depending entirely on commercial conditions.

The Pylorus

There is a valve at the exit of the stomach which is known as the **pyloric valve**. This valve controls the volume which leaves the stomach after the gastric juices have done their work on the food or material which has been swallowed. Liquids usually pass through the pyloric valve with priority over the bolus. The pyloric valve has glands which secrete an alkaline liquid containing pepsin, as well as a substance which acts as a chemical medium to stimulate the gastric juices. This substance does not go into the stomach but is taken into the bloodstream which carries it to the gastric glands, stimulating them to secrete. The effect of this activity is not a usual reflex caused by nerves, but the stimulation of one organ by chemical substances produced in another.

It must be remembered that the hormone secreted by the pyloric glands is mostly pepsin and hydrochloric acid. This same combination is used inside the stomach to break down and liquefy solid proteins. The importance of this pyloric gland secretion is therefore very apparent in the fact that no solid protein of any kind can be utilized in the process of digestion, but must be liquefied. Thus, nature has provided an extra margin of safety to insure the complete liquefaction of proteins which were not liquefied in the stomach.

The Liver

At the top of the ascending colon where it curves to the right on the chart (curves to left in the body) is the area marked **liver**. This curve is known as the **Hepatic** (or Liver) **Flexure**, and is located immediately over the liver. The liver is composed of the right lobe and the left lobe, the right lobe being by far the greater and larger of the two.

The liver is the largest gland in the body and is the organ carrying on the most active and extensive operation in the anatomy. Everything that goes down the throat, in the form of food or otherwise, and every beverage that we drink, sip or pour down our throat must pass through, in more or less liquid form,the 25 feet of small intestine. The small intestine is equipped with millions of tiny organs like suction cups, called villi, which avidly grab every molecule that can be collected from the material inside the small intestine and pass these molecules to the surrounding blood vessels. The blood in these vessels instantly takes these molecules to the liver where they are split up into their component atoms. The segregated atoms are then catalogued and assigned to other atoms which, in turn, form new molecules of the kind the body calls for and which the cells and tissues of the body can use.

Thus, it is useless to eat such things as "a complete protein" with the expectation and the false assurance that this complete protein will be used by the body. The so-called complete protein must first be emulsified into a heterogenous mass called chyme and mixed with everything else in the small intestine. In such a state, all molecules in the chyme, whatever they happen to

FRONT SURFACE OF LIVER

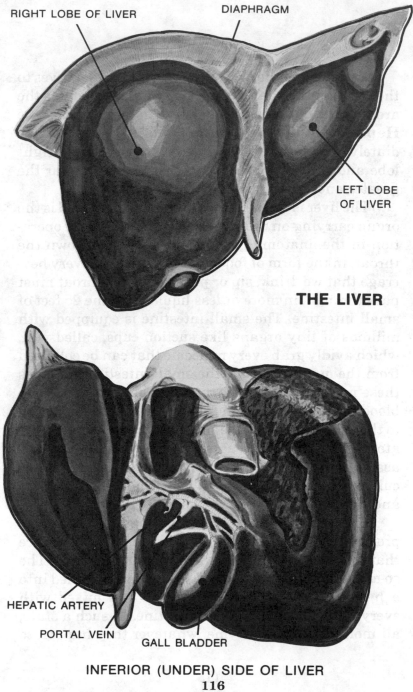

RIGHT LOBE OF LIVER

DIAPHRAGM

LEFT LOBE OF LIVER

THE LIVER

HEPATIC ARTERY

PORTAL VEIN

GALL BLADDER

INFERIOR (UNDER) SIDE OF LIVER

116

be, are gathered by the villi and passed by the blood stream to the liver.

What was originally sugar and starch is likewise broken down into their respective molecules and these, in turn, are disintegrated into the separate atoms composing them and reassembled to form glucose. This is then converted into glycogen and stored for reconversion into glucose, which can be released into the circulating blood for delivery where it is needed. Glucose is a form of sugar found in blood, in lymph, and is present in many fruits, such as grape-sugar, etc. Glycogen is a tasteless carbohydrate related to dextrin and starch.

The liver is naturally involved in the collection of the various molecules composing the many vitamins necessary for our well-being. Consider the many atoms which enter into the composition of vitamins. Here are a few chosen at random:

C = Carbon,   H = Hydrogen,   O = Oxygen
Cl = Chlorine,   N = Nitrogen,   S = Sulphur

Vitamin A = C_{20}, H_{29}, HO

Vitamin B_1 Thiamin = $C_{12}, H_{17}, ClN_4, OS$

B_2 Riboflavin = C_{17}, H_{20}, N_4, O_6

Vitamin B_6 = C_8, H_{11}, NO_3

Vitamin C = C_6, H_8, O_6

Vitamin D = C_{28}, H_{43}, OH

Vitamin E - a/tocopherol = C_{29}, H_{50}

Vitamin E = b/ & y/tocopherol = C_{28}, H_{48}, O_2

Vitamin K = C_{31}, H_{46}, O_2

The vitamin department of the liver cannot utilize any vitamins as a whole, composite substance. The nutritional activities of the body do not function this way. The volume of each vitamin in grams is so microscopic that only a miraculous computerized system, working within the anatomy in a most mysterious manner, could have any more effect on a 150 -or 200-pound body than on the body of a child. One pound of peeled bananas, for example, contains on an average, less than one-quarter of a milligram of Vitamin B_1 (Thiamin) and only about 0.29 milligrams of Riboflavin. Now realize that there are 28,350 milligrams in one ounce and 453,370 milligrams in one-pound weight. Cauliflower has only one-half a milligram each of Thiamin and Riboflavin per one-pound weight.

Obviously, if we eat mostly raw vegetables and fruits, nuts, sprouted seeds, plus raw vegetables juices, we can get all the vitamins the body needs. I have never taken any vitamins as I get all that my body needs by keeping my colon clean and eating this type of food. I have never found myself deficient in vitamins. Why? The atoms which my liver needs to make up whatever vitamins my system requires are obtained from the raw food I eat, plus the juices I drink.

When I was a young fellow, before I knew any better, I ate what most Scottish people ate: porridge with milk and sugar, lots of starches such as scones, and cookies such as Singing Hinnies made of starch and sugar. This caused my liver to become greatly disturbed, and it reacted accordingly. When I drank lots of carrot juice, I was rewarded with a complete recovery; however, the accumulated bile could not be eliminated through my clogged-up colon fast enough and it was eliminated through the pores of my skin. Everybody thought I had contracted jaundice, but after a few months it cleared and my skin was better than ever. Does it surprise you that I try to live as closely as possible to what nature dictates? Don't envy me, go thou and do likewise.

A very important activity of the liver is the generation of bile. After the bile is generated it is stored in the gall bladder to be released into the duodenum, or second stomach, whenever anything passes through it from the stomach. We will be discussing the role of the bile in our next chapter. Suffice it here to say that bile is involved in the digestion and absorption of fats.

The liver is greatly concerned with preventing blood-clotting. As vitamin K is known to prevent hemorrhage, you should appreciate the work involved in combining the vitamin K formula listed in a preceding paragraph. Just think, gathering together 31 carbon atoms, 46 hydrogen atoms and 2 oxygen atoms to form the Vitamin K molecules — thousands of which will be needed to prevent your blood from clotting. It staggers the imagination! If you will nourish your body properly, keep your colon clean and your mind elevated, your liver will take care of you.

Other functions of the liver are concerned with fat and protein metabolism. The liver is a detoxifying agent and a blood reservoir. It breaks down the hemoglobin of the red cells which have already served their purpose, and also stores copper, iron, and other trace elements for instant use when needed.

Be careful of your liver. If it breaks down beyond repair, you will be finished with your body and will have to step out of it forever.

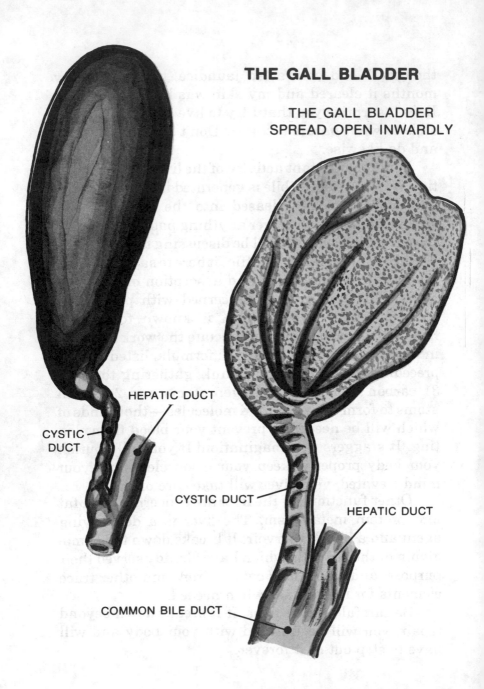

THE GALL BLADDER

THE GALL BLADDER
SPREAD OPEN INWARDLY

HEPATIC DUCT

CYSTIC
DUCT

CYSTIC DUCT

HEPATIC DUCT

COMMON BILE DUCT

It is harmful and dangerous to neglect to care for the condition of the colon. Parasitical interference with any of the functions of the body, and of the liver in particular, is the cause of most ailments and physical afflictions. It is for this reason that one makes no mistake in taking a series of colon irrigations annually, unfailingly, as long as there is life in the body — particularly if one eats orthodox foods prepared in the orthodox manner.

The Gall Bladder

The **gall bladder** is a bulbous sack attached to the underside of the liver in order to serve as storage for the bile secreted by the liver.

Bile is an important element in the process of digestion as it is mainly involved in the digestion of fats. Bile helps in the digestive processes by neutralizing the acid chyme which passes through the duodenum from the stomach by emulsifying fats. It also promotes peristalsis, the absorption of elements in the body, by helping to prevent putrefaction.

The bile is composed of certain acids which form an intimately related group of natural products. While the bile acids occur free to some extent, they are usually combined with glycine or taurine (as in glycocholic acid and taurocholic acid) which results from the break down of proteins. Two of the better known bile acids are cholic and lithocholic.

Cholesterin (cholesterol) is a white, fatty, crystalline alcohol, tasteless and without odor, found abundantly in the tissue of nerves; it is also present in bile and in gall stones. As it contains no nitrogen, it is not a

121

part of protein. Lecithin and cholesterin usually are found together, which indicates a physiological aspect to their function.

I should deviate here for a moment to relate the interesting result of using Cleaver's herb with which both gall stones and kidney stones have been completely dissolved. A gall stone about 10 millimeters (about three-eighths of an inch) in diameter was placed in a test tube which was then filled with a teaspoonful of Cleaver's herb steeped in a cup of hot, just short of boiling, distilled water. Within 48 hours there was no trace of the stone to be seen. This has been repeated a number of times with similar results, leading to the correct conclusion that by the use of a cup of Cleaver's tea three or four times a day, coupled with colon irrigations, it is possible for such stones to be dissolved and the bile duct cleared.

The gall bladder is an extremely important organ in the body. To remove it only results in the development of subsequent difficulties in digesting food properly.

The Pancreas

The **pancreas** is a long, narrow gland of internal and external secretion. It stretches from the spleen to a wee bit higher than the middle of the semi-circular bend of the duodenum. Its main duct joins the duct of the gall bladder, emptying into the duodenum. The pancreas is a compound tubular gland like the salivary glands in the mouth.

The pancreas is one of the most active glands in

the system. Everything that goes through the duodenum requires some of the digestive juices produced in the pancreas. Pancreatic juice contains digestive enzymes and is alkaline in its reaction, serving to establish the right conditions for the intestinal enzymes to do their work in the small intestine.

Towards the middle of the pancreas there is a group of glands of internal secretion, known as the islands of langerhans, which produce insulin, the hormone which regulates the metabolism of sugar (the blood sugar level) and other carbohydrates. When the body is toxic and the colon is afflicted with fermentation and putrefaction, these glands are unable to produce this insulin, causing an intolerance of sugar by the body. Under these circumstances the volume of sugar is increased in the blood and is discharged into the kidneys. This condition is called sugar diabetes or diabetes mellitus. Many people so afflicted have found that the cleansing of the colon by means of a series of colon irrigations, coupled with a complete change of diet of fresh, raw vegetable and fruit juices, raw vegetables and fruits, and nuts and sprouted seeds, has made it possible for them to avoid the further use of manufactured insulin. In fact, they found they derived much benefit from drinking one or two pints, every day, of the combination of carrot, celery, string bean and brussel sprout juice as indicated in my book, *Fresh Vegetable and Fruit Juices*.

The pancreas is a very important gland in our body and we should give to it the full complement of respect

THE PANCREAS

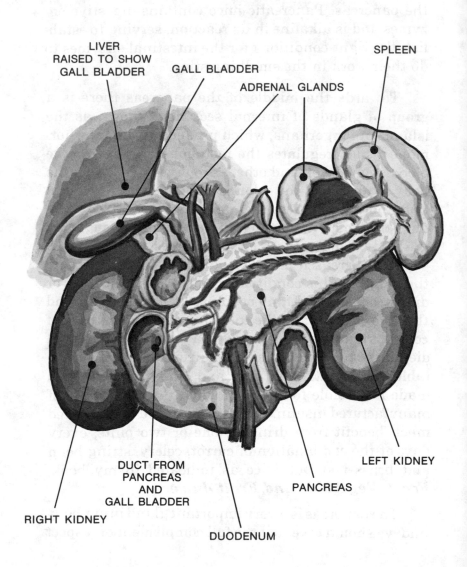

LIVER
RAISED TO SHOW
GALL BLADDER

GALL BLADDER

ADRENAL GLANDS

SPLEEN

DUCT FROM
PANCREAS
AND
GALL BLADDER

RIGHT KIDNEY

DUODENUM

PANCREAS

LEFT KIDNEY

which it deserves if we wish to attain any degree of perfect, vibrant health. The first place to begin is with your colon.

Strange, is it not, that we human beings have to be knocked flat before we will listen to the wisdom with which God Almighty has endowed us. The summing up of the whole duty of man is to learn what is true, in order to do what is right.

The Spleen

The **spleen** is an organ lying on the left side of the body inside the lower ribs. It is connected to the stomach by the gastro-splenic ligament and to the left kidney by the kidney ligament. The spleen is composed largely of loose, adenoid tissue known as the splenic pulp.

It has its own inherent mechanism by means of which it expands and contracts, swelling up somewhat during the digestion of food. It is a large blood-filter placed on the main stream of blood vessels known as the splenic-lienal artery. Among its many functions is the removal of used-up, dead, red blood corpuscles from the blood, as well as any bacteria and other waste matter which might be present. The spleen also produces antibiotics.

After conception and during the development of the fetus, the spleen manufactures blood cells and red blood corpuscles, stores these, and delivers them into the blood stream as is necessary.

There are some functions of the spleen which have

THE SPLEEN

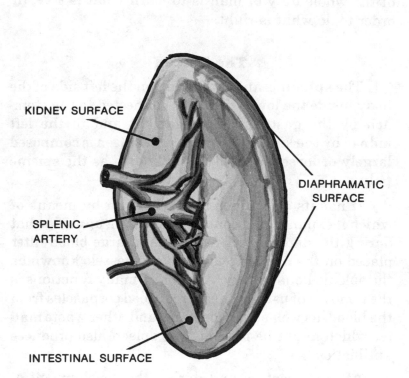

KIDNEY SURFACE

DIAPHRAMATIC SURFACE

SPLENIC ARTERY

INTESTINAL SURFACE

not yet been observed. Of one thing we are certain, constipation has a definite depressing effect on the spleen, which affects digestion. Undoubtedly the reason for this is that constipation, like any other affliction of the colon, creates a toxic state which reacts on the entire system. To help keep the spleen in top condition it is a good principle to maintain a regular yearly schedule of colon irrigations and to use **high** enemas whenever necessary.

The difference between a plain enema and a **high** enema is the length of the colon tube used. When purchasing an enema bag, a short, hard rubber or plastic tube accompanies it. However, for a **high** enema we use a 30-inch colon or rectal tube made of soft, pliable, good quality rubber; this is attached to the short, hard tube which comes with the enema bag. When this 30-inch tube is lubricated with a suitable lubricant jelly, it is easily inserted in the anus after the bag has been filled with the necessary warm water. Once the descending colon has been cleared by previous cleansings, the tube can be inserted two or three inches at a time, reaching across the transverse colon and thereby achieving a satisfactory high enema.

The Appendix

Proceeding up to the right of the cecum we meet the **appendix**, technically known as the vermiform appendix. The length of the appendix may be anywhere between one inch and six, or in rare cases even eight inches long. The usual length is about three inches.

Through its entire center is a channel surrounded

by an infinite number of glands which leads right into the cecum. The appendix is under the general control of the hypothalamus which, among all its other functions, is charged with the protection of the human body. The appendix is an organ, or better expressed as a gland, which has received only a fraction of the interest and attention it should have since it was first created by Almighty God who knew exactly why He placed it there. I want you to particularly notice the cross-section picture of the appendix, illustrated in this chapter, showing the infinite number of glands it contains. This picture, or course, is greatly magnified.

Why do you suppose the Creator went to the trouble to place the appendix right in that particular spot? Let me tell you. The appendix generates and secretes a powerful **germicidal** fluid which is automatically injected into the cecum only when the waste matter coming from the small intestine through the ileo-cecal valve is potentially harmful to the welfare of the individual.

A medical dictionary I have brushes off the importance of the appendix by describing it simply as "the small blind gut projecting from the cecum." As a matter of fact, the appendix is the "Watchman on the Tower" so to speak; or in other words, it is the first line of defense located where the residue from digestion of food leaves the small intestine and enters the colon through the ileo-cecal valve. When healthy and in good working order, the appendix is alerted and injects into the cecum its germicidal fluid which neutralizes any residue that could in any way interfere with the proper

THE APPENDIX

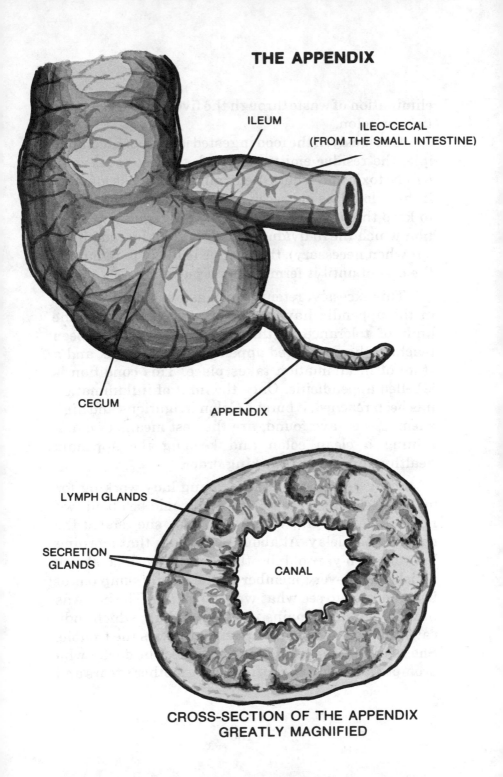

ILEUM

ILEO-CECAL
(FROM THE SMALL INTESTINE)

CECUM

APPENDIX

LYMPH GLANDS

SECRETION
GLANDS

CANAL

CROSS-SECTION OF THE APPENDIX
GREATLY MAGNIFIED

elimination of waste through the five feet of large intestine, or colon.

Obviously, if the food ingested is toxic or incompatible, the residue emitted through the ileo-cecal valve will be toxic and require neutralizaton. In like manner, if the colon does not receive the attention it must have to keep the waste matter moving out regularly (attention which the individual must give to it by washing it out when necessary), the residue is likely to remain in the cecum until it ferments and putrefies.

This excessive retention of waste eventually results in the appendix having to work overtime. When the limit of tolerance in this overtime work has been reached, the poor, tired appendix becomes sick and a state of inflammation takes place. This condition is labelled appendicitis. Once the limit of inflammation has been reached, it bursts. Colon irrigations and high enemas, we have found, are the best means of maintaining a clean colon and keeping the appendix healthy and in good working order.

Many years ago, I had a young lady working for me who telephoned to tell me she would be about two hours late for work. When she came, she related the cause of her delay. At about two o'clock that morning her fourteen-year-old brother awoke with a shriek which made every member of the family jump out of bed and rush to see what was the matter. The boy was having agonizing pains in his right loin, which indicated to his mother that appendicitis was the trouble. She rushed to the telephone and called the doctor who promptly arrived. He confirmed the mother's fears and ordered the boy immediately to the hospital.

As soon as the doctor left, the boy's sister (my secretary) took out her enema bag and gave the boy a high enema every half hour, for four hours. When the ambulance arrived, the intern examined the boy and said there was no need to take him to the hospital as he seemed to be getting along very well. The boy rested all that day and was back in school the following day.

Unfortunately, the germicidal fluid of the appendix does not destroy either worms or their eggs; thus, under conditions favorable for the development of a colony of worms, these can nest and propagate in the bottom of the cecum, causing the V-shape to form which is visible in an X ray.

Any disturbance of the appendix or of its performance is the direct result of toxic residue emanating from the small intestine as a result of the ingestion of the wrong kinds of foods and beverages which has become a habit whenever appetite led the way to the refrigerator, the dining table or to the coffee house. We just cannot escape this tragic state of affairs as long as we eat to satisfy the mind and the palate instead of considering, "What does my body **need**?"

It has been very gratifying to me that my books *Become Younger, Fresh Vegetable and Fruit Juices,* and *Guide to Diet and Salads* have been consistently in demand since I first published them, and today they are in greater demand than ever. The thousands of letters which I have received — and am still receiving from the world over — confirm the fact that the **Walker Program** outlined in these books has been of value and effect for everyone who followed it through.

This is not intended as a "plug" for my books. I mention this because so many people ask, "What can I do to be saved from these afflictions?" And after having been told to purchase and **study** my books, putting into practice the natural principles outlined therein, they eventually write — and even telephone — to tell me what wonderful results they had.

It all boils down to this: Eat as much raw food as possible, drink fresh raw vegetable and fruit juices, drink at least two pints of **distilled water** every day, and **never** neglect giving attention to the colon. Take high enemas whenever needed (they are **not** habit-forming) and never hesitate to have some colon irrigations — twice a year if necessary — every year as long as you live. Your appendix will appreciate it —every part of your anatomy will appreciate it!— and you may avoid that horrible period of premature senility, as well as enjoy a comfortable, peaceful, healthy old age.

Don't look behind! Keep your sights on the present and the future. The past is history; your future is ahead of you. See that you make it well worthwhile.

One last word: Don't part with or lose your appendix. It would be very much like killing the goose that lays the golden egg. If your appendix has already been amputated, make the best of it by watching your diet and your colon even more meticulously.

Your Adrenal Glands

The **adrenal glands** are sometimes called the

supra-renals, derived from the archaic "reins" for kidneys. In the book of Isaiah, chapter 11, verse 5 we read, *"Faithfulness [shall be] the girdle of His reins,"* and several other such expressions.

The adrenal glands are like a hat on the top of each kidney, each gland consisting of two distinct sections: the center part called the medulla and the outer part the cortex. The medulla stems from the nerves which are the source of the sympathetic nerve system, thereby directly connecting it with the rest of the body. The medulla also secretes the hormone epinephrine. With the possible exception of the thyroid gland, the adrenals have a richer supply of blood than any other organ of relative size in the body. *See pg. 124 & 156.*

The cortex with its hormones is essential to life. If there should happen to be a deficiency of these hormones, a disturbance of the fluid and of the electrolyte balance in the system will follow. These hormones are involved to a very important extent in the metabolism of protein, fats and carbohydrates. Emotional excitement, intense muscular exertion, cold, pain, and shock are all conditions of stress which these hormones enable the individual to meet as occasion arises. Failure of the adrenals to produce these hormones will also reduce the ability of the body to resist infection.

Cortisone is a preparation manufactured with the intent to duplicate the effect of this hormone and has in some instances proved effective; however, the side-effects in far too many cases have been very harmful to the victim of its use. Personally, from my own observation of some of these side-effects, I would not under any circumstances subject my body to its use.

The cortex is under the control of the pituitary gland and, in addition, the two have a reciprocal cooperative function. Obviously, what will affect one gland will also have a similar effect on the other. Because of their close proximity, a radical disturbance of the kidneys automatically disturbs the adrenals, but the effect of fermentation and putrefaction in the colon has a more constant negative effect on both the adrenals and the pituitary. A poor colon condition in every way can harm the rest of the body and the important glands in particular.

As stated above, the medulla produces the hormone epinephrine. This hormone is also manufactured for injection into the bloodstream, causing acceleration of the heart and constriction of the blood vessels, thus raising the blood pressure. Another effect is on the liver, releasing sugar which, in turn, raises the level of sugar in the blood. The hormone adrenalin is also secreted by the adrenals and differs so very little from the epinephrine that its formula makes an interesting study. Epinephrine is composed of $C_{10}H_{13}NO_3$ plus $\frac{1}{2}H_2O$, while the formula for adrenalin is $C_9H_{13}NO_3$. Notice that the former has just one atom more of C (carbon) than adrenalin. They both have more or less similar effects on the system. When these hormones have been injected into the spinal cord the blood pressure rises more than 100% by the time the hypodermic needle is removed.

In laboratory tests, the action of adrenal extracts (adrenalin) on muscle always reflects the effect of stimulating the nerves of the sympathetic nerve system supplying the muscle. Obviously, the secretion of the adrenalin hormone in the adrenal glands has a direct effect on the nervous system of the body. Undue stress in our work or other phases of our lives would cause the excessive production of adrenalin in the body, increasing nervous tension.

Injections of adrenalin in patients afflicted with Addison's disease have not had permanent results because the injections soon lose their effect. This is understandable when we consider the multiplicity of effects resulting from this affliction: marked emaciation, progressive anemia, low blood pressure, gastrointestinal disturbance and extreme debility. Although this is a chronic and frequently fatal malady, we have known victims who, considering everything else of no avail, decided to try a drastic cleansing program by means of many weeks of colon irrigations, an ample intake of fresh raw vegetable and fruit juices, fresh raw vegetables, fruits, nuts and sprouted seeds, and found it to be very beneficial.

In the final analysis there is no question that the natural course of the use by the body of its adrenal secretions is intended by Nature to keep the blood pure and active, provided the individual does his share to keep the body clean and properly nourished. The tone of the muscles is dependent on the adrenal secretions; without them, debility is bound to follow. These secretions are also essential because of their anti-toxic effect on toxins in the body as a result of metabolism.

The adrenal glands have a very definite and strong effect on the reproductive organs. To allow the mind to become obsessed with sex has a direct malevolent effect on the adrenals, resulting in what we would call a pornographic mental aberration. Masturbation is one of these means by which this state of mind may develop; other sex deviations have similar effects.

It is wise to keep both the mind and the colon clean.

Chapter 8.
The Reproductive Organs And Their Effect On The Colon

The **genitals** are the reproductive organs. Generally, the physical, mental and spiritual care and use of these incredibly wonderful organs of reproduction are completely blanketed by the senses.

It is a perfectly normal and natural function of every specie to reproduce in order that they should not become extinct. However, the excessive use and abuse of these organs is directly responsible for many afflictions of the human race.

Appetite, in every form and respect, is one of man's most insidious enemies. Hunger is the body's call for food, but an excessive appetite becomes a vice which usually results in drastic and unforeseen afflictions when it is used and indulged in to excess.

While discussing the appetite, it is important to consider the effect of food on the system. Excessive use of hot condiments results in over-stimulation of the digestive system which, in turn, affects the kidneys and the genitals around them. The stimulation of the genitals by the use of hot peppers and the like is notorious, as is the excessive consumption of heavy meats, such as the flesh of animals.

Many years ago a noted health lecturer who prided himself on his physique and his manly vigor, having copiously eaten flesh all his life, decided that perhaps the **Walker Program** might have some merits. He sampled the program for about two years, after which he returned to his former eating habits, claiming that while it **did** effectively improve his health, the program had the tendency to slow down his sexual proclivities.

Anything that we put into our system that stimulates sex desire and activity can automatically have a negative, degenerating effect on the cells and tissues of the brain. This, as a general rule, has the tendency to cause the individual to become a deviate, given to considerable departure from the norms of behavior in society.

Male Organs: the Testes

The **testis** (plural is testes or testicles) is the male genital or reproductive gland corresponding to the ovary in the female. It produces the spermatozoa. The spermatozoa, or sperm, has the function of fertilizing the egg. It is relatively small in relation to the egg. Being a live organism, it is more or less capable of active, spontaneous movement by which it approaches or enters the egg. It is discharged in a gelatinous fluid known as the semen.

When one considers that the period of reproducing a single orgasm or discharge of the semen requires an average of 35 days, it can readily be appreciated why the excessive discharge of this semen causes weakness, and when deliberately exercised by an adult may cause premature loss of the ability to function sexually. All

THE TESTICLES

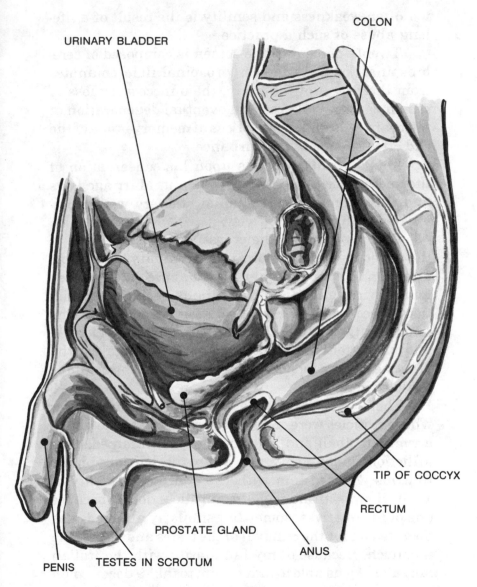

COLON

URINARY BLADDER

TIP OF COCCYX

RECTUM

ANUS

PROSTATE GLAND

PENIS

TESTES IN SCROTUM

CROSS SECTION OF LOWER PELVIC REGION

too often weakness and senility is the result of a life-long abuse of such a practice.

Twenty percent of the semen is composed of cerebrospinal fluid. As the cerebrospinal fluid emanates from the region of the brain, the unnecessary loss of semen causes weakness and eventual degeneration of the brain cells and tissues. Loss of memory is one of the end-effects of such a disturbance.

Man's virility depends upon his conservation of the sperm, not his ability to waste it. Marriage laws and the commandment against adultery were promulgated with this end in view.

If you will study the cross-section illustration of the pelvic region and look at the proximity of the prostate gland to the rectum, you will appreciate the need for colon irrigations to prevent the excessive accumulation of feces and other waste matter in the region of the anus and the rectum. Once this area becomes clogged and its contents magnified, the pressure against the prostate can, and usually does, cause either prostate or testicle trouble.

There comes to mind a case of an Italian laborer whose testicles were enlarged very nearly to the size of a rugby football and his prostate also inflamed. This affliction, undoubtedly, was due to the delicious pizzas that his wife fed him with the addition of plenty of Vino. He was afraid to go to a medical doctor because one of his relatives, somewhat similarly afflicted, was operated on for the removal of the testes and he became a eunuch. Because of my familiarity with the Italian language I was able to induce him to take a dozen colon irrigations. In the course of two or three months he appeared on his own volition for another dozen irrigations. In about 18 months his testicles were almost normal and his prostate trouble had vanished.

The Prostate Gland

The word **prostate** in anatomical language is derived from the Greek "prostates," which means "one who stands before." The **prostate gland**, located between the rectum and the neck of the urinary bladder in the male, is partly muscular and partly glandular. It discharges a viscid, opalescent secretion into ducts leading to the floor of the urethra. The urethra is the canal which carries the urine from the bladder and also serves as the genital duct.

The strategic location of the prostate between the urinary bladder and the rectum necessitates giving meticulous attention to everything that man puts into his system. Between the fermenting and putrefacting waste matter in the colon, on the one hand, and the many insidious elements which can find their way into the kidneys and the urinary bladder, on the other hand, we have the perfect set-up for two vicious ailments to which the prostate is an easy victim: namely, inflammation and cancer.

Inflammation can so restrict the urethra that urination may be painful. When the condition is aggravated, the emptying of the bladder may not be possible. This condition is known as prostatitis.

The prostate gland is also an easy prey to cancer if internal cleanliness is not practiced meticulously.

Deep resentments, stress, worry, anger, fear and the multiplicity of similar attitudes are definite contributing factors which predispose the prostate gland to ailments and disease.

We had a young friend in his mid-thirties, with three children, who was filled with fear lest he fail to take proper care of his family financially. He worked hard, much too hard, and at too long a stretch at a time. He was always worrying, yet tried to keep his fears and worries from becoming apparent to others, particularly to his wife. He tried to be meticulous about eating correct food and generally strived to take good care of himself, under the circumstances. All this was of no avail. He developed inflammation of the prostate which turned into cancer. His wife insisted that he go to the hospital, which he did very much against his wishes and better judgment. He left the hospital for his final eternal home while his widow was left to take care of what was left of his body. The doctors said he died of cancer. I say he died as a result of his negative frame of mind. Even colon irrigations cannot overcome a negative state of mind. How very true it is that, "As a man thinketh, so is he."

Colon irrigations are the first line of defense for the prostate in particular, as they prevent the accumulation of waste matter and feces which can clog up the rectum. This is a matter far too serious and important to pass over lightly. One cannot imagine the vast ramifications of afflictions, ailments and diseases which can eventually result from neglecting to keep the colon clean and bowel movements regular. This insistence is not fanaticism; it is good, common sense. When this matter is neglected and the point of no return is reached, it is too late to wish that it had been taken care of years ago. Failure to practice prevention may turn out to be lethal.

What is probably the greatest and most insidious contributing factor to any kind of prostate trouble is the unnatural use of the sex organs, such as masturbation and homosexual practices. It takes from 10 to 25 years for such trouble to manifest itself. By that time, the point of no return may have been reached. Such deviate practices afflict the brain area almost more than any other part of the body because of the cerebro-spinal fluid involvment.

Female Organs — The Uterus

The **uterus** is the female organ of reproduction. It is more than that, however, as it is intimately involved with the life-long problems of the female to such an extent that it can, and usually does, affect the entire domestic environment.

Generally speaking, the troubles of a woman who is not married never end, but when a woman gets married her troubles are multiplied!

Perhaps the least known cause of one of woman's greatest handicaps, **fatigue** (constant weariness, inability to "catch up" with insufficient sleep), is the loss of her **tonsils**. This fact is not generally recognized, yet it is proven daily. Nevertheless, children — and frequently adults —are still subjected to the needless loss of these two vital little organs which have a vast and a devastating effect on the entire life of the individual. And please bear in mind that males are not in the least more resistant to this evil than females.

As already explained in a preceding chapter on the subject of **tonsils**, it is rarely necessary to remove them. Their inflamed or diseased condition is a warning that there is far too much toxicity in the body for the system to overcome without serious consequences. Instead of removing the tonsils, a series of colon irrigations would help to remove the corruption in the body, which manifested itself in afflicted tonsils.

A woman who has had her tonsils removed, who has six children whose tonsils have likewise been removed, has multiplied her share of troubles sixfold; namely, her own and those of each of her children. Be sure to study the chapter of this book entitled **Connective Tissue And Vitamin C**.

In discussing the physical appearance of the uterus, we find that it is a single, thick-walled, muscular, hollow organ, which is more or less pear-shaped. The urinary bladder is in front of it and the rectum and sigmoid flexure of the descending colon are behind it.

Now examine the two pictures of the colon, the illustration of the **normal colon** and the one showing the colon filled with corruption and waste impactions. Imagine the rectum and the sigmoid flexure bloated with solid fecal matter behind the uterus, and the urinary bladder filled to capacity because time has not been taken to empty it. The uterus is squeezed between these two bloated organs! Is it surprising that there are so many instances of a prolapsed uterus? It would be

THE UTERUS

SANDWICHED BETWEEN THE RECTUM AND THE URINARY BLADDER

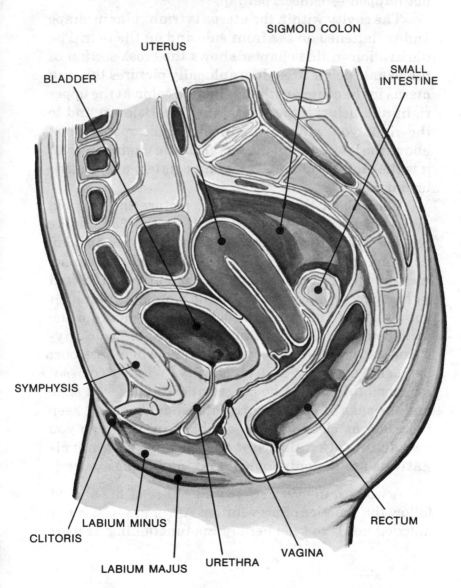

BLADDER

UTERUS

SIGMOID COLON

SMALL INTESTINE

SYMPHYSIS

LABIUM MINUS

CLITORIS

LABIUM MAJUS

URETHRA

VAGINA

RECTUM

indeed very surprising if something more serious does not happen — cancer, perhaps?

The cavity within the uterus is triangular in shape and is flattened on the front side and on the rear. The illustration in this chapter shows the cross-section of the female pelvic area. It graphically pictures the long uterus in the center, with the sigmoid colon at the upper right and below it the small intestine. Below it and to the right you will see the inside of the rectum; just above the lower part of the rectum is the vagina, next to it is the urethral channel and immediately above is the urinary bladder.

Looking at this illustration, picture the sigmoid and the rectum distended with the accumulative residue of a lifetime of incomplete evacuations. In addition, imagine yourself with the bladder filled to capacity and you are unable to get to the bathroom to void right away. What happens to the womb or uterus? If you happen to be pregnant, what punishment for the child being developed within, utterly unable to do **anything** except patiently await the time when he is born deficient, mentally and physically. What a colossal responsibility it is to be pregnant! For your own sake and the sake of your unborn child should you not keep the colon as clean as you possibly can! How can you best do that? Certainly **not** by laxatives! **Colon irrigations** are the only logical and intelligent answer!

A woman in every stage and phase of life should follow the practice of prevention. A woman who is not married needs to keep her organs functioning as near

146

to perfection as possible in order to prevent the unavoidable consequences of neglect. A woman's greatest tragedy is to look old and haggard at 30, 40 and 50 years of age. This state is not necessary if she will learn to eradicate from her mind and consciousness every vestige of resentment and take things as they come, remembering that the evil might be worse. Avoid becoming jealous, angry and vindictive, and put **all** negative thoughts and feelings in the waste basket. That's where they belong! Don't ever blame anyone on earth except Eve for eating the forbidden fruit and bringing all troubles upon womankind. Be happy, joyous and enthusiastic! It helps!

I should add a few words about smoking, which is one of the most degenerating and degrading practices to which so many women have become addicted. If you think that smoking is glamorous, you are worse than foolish. If you think that smoking "quiets your nerves," you are bordering on idiocy. The most harmful habit that a woman can acquire is smoking. She becomes a nicotine addict. Why? Because a woman needs pure blood, and one of the life-sources of the blood is the air which is breathed into the lungs. The blood extracts the oxygen from the air for the sustenance and cleansing of the cells and tissues of the body and extracts nitrogen for the regeneration of amino acids composing the protein in the system. Tobacco smoke clogs up the little grape-like bunches of air-sacs in the lungs, making it impossible for them to make full use of clean air. Just as it is impossible to smoke without inhaling, it is impossible to breathe pure air in a smoke-filled room.

MAMMARY GLAND

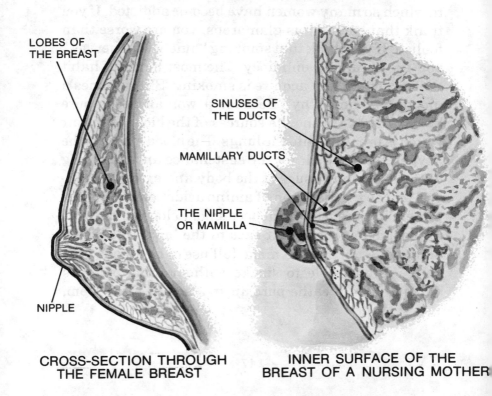

LOBES OF
THE BREAST

SINUSES OF
THE DUCTS

MAMILLARY DUCTS

THE NIPPLE
OR MAMILLA

NIPPLE

CROSS-SECTION THROUGH
THE FEMALE BREAST

INNER SURFACE OF THE
BREAST OF A NURSING MOTHER

Even if a person does not smoke, breathing smoke-polluted air has a similar effect on the system. If women could just take a peek in some of the "hidden" sections of hospitals specializing in the treatment of cancer, they could see men and women with no noses, or mouths, or anything left of the lower part of their faces, because it has been all eaten away by cancer caused by tabacco smoke. If you envy such people and you don't care what you look like, then, dear sister, go ahead and smoke all you want!

Smoking by women also has a direct effect on the reproductive organs, frequently causing premature menopause with its concomitant pains and discomforts. Anything that interferes with Nature's processes results in a disruption of the comforts of life.

Failure to keep the urinary bladder voided as promptly as possible, while the sigmoid and the rectum are filled with fermentation and putrefaction, can result in many of the menstrual troubles with which girls and women are frequently afflicted. Colon irrigations can save you so much trouble!

The Mammary Glands

The woman's breast, known as the **mammary glands**, is inextricably connected and related to her reproductive system. The mammary glands, however, have a far wider relationship which involves participation in the functions and activities of other glands such as the pituitary gland, the parathyroid, the adrenal glands, and of course, very strongly, the ovaries. Also the influence of the mammary glands on the tonsils is tremendous. This regulating and balancing effect naturally involves the welfare of the entire system, not in the least the psychological, the emotional and the spiritual phases of a woman's everyday life.

Obviously, when this particular sacculation of the colon which relates to the mammary glands is allowed to accumulate an excessive volume of fecal and other waste matter, fermenting and putrefying, the mammary glands will relay this condition to the other glands, and an unaccountable disturbance will arise which gives a woman the epithet of being unstable and fickle.

As a matter of fact, when a woman is in as nearly a perfect health condition as is possible for her to be in this day and generation, she finds her intuitive faculties quite keen and alert. On the other hand, when the colon has been neglected for a lifetime, better instincts are dimmed and the mind leans toward self-pity, which often leads to such perversions as lesbianism. This is particularly the case when the tonsils have been removed.

The pituitary gland, as we have seen in a preceding chapter, has administrative rulership over the nerves. We have frequently noticed from X rays of the colon that, while the cecum sacculation which denotes the connection with the pituitary seems to be in order, the sacculation relating to the mammary glands indicates a disturbance. This is reflected in a nervous condition in women and can disappear after a series of colon irrigations have been administered.

In the relationship of the mammary glands to the

adrenals and the parathyroid, there could be a disturbance of fat metabolism as well as the possible inception of tumors. A worse disturbance could arise from the lymphatic system which could express itself as lumps in the breast. Such disturbances have satisfactorily responded to the cleansing of the colon by a series of colon irrigations.

The mammary glands have much to do with the regulation of menstruation. Irregularities in this area are all too frequently related to the impacted condition of the colon. The accompanying picture, copied from an X ray which was made of the colon of a 36-year-old lady, indicates how seriously the balance and the regularity of the female anatomy and its functions can be affected. In this particular case, note the inverted "V" at the bottom of the ascending colon, indicating the presence of worms. At the other end of the colon, notice how impacted the rectum is with waste matter. This indicates gross neglect on her part to respond to the call of the bowel. It also points out the harm that the weight of this mass would have on the uterus and the urinary bladder, all of which would result in the disturbance of the menstrual process.

It is bad enough that a man would neglect to keep his colon clean causing a bloated rectum to give him prostate trouble, but a woman has far more and varied troubles which she could and **must** prevent if she expects to bypass the many afflictions which befall women.

Do not think for one moment that colon irrigations

ABNORMAL COLON OF A 36-YEAR-OLD WOMAN

From X-Ray of Colon of Mrs. R.G. - Los Angeles.

REMARKS: Patient was a typical consumer of Meat and Starches. This Colon is more or less characteristic of those of consumers of mixed-cooked foods, using the average amount of meat and starches.

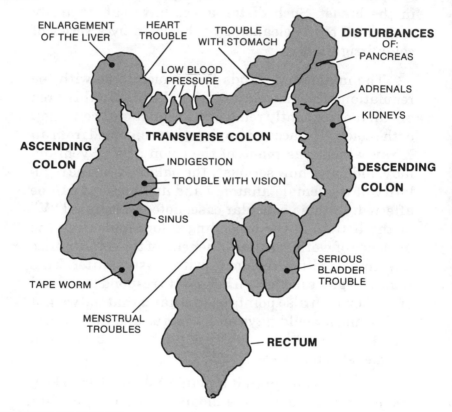

URINALYSIS INDICATIONS:

UREA from Kidneys: 3.1 grams per 1000 c.c. *(0.3%)*. *(Normal - 30 to 35 grams.)*

OXALIC ACID CRYSTALS: Too many to count, *(Indicating ingestion of cooked Spinach or Rhubarb - Raw Spinach does not leave this residue of crystals.)*

TOTAL SOLIDS: 80.6 grams per 1000 c.c. *(Normal - 40-50 gr.) (Indicating inefficiency of Kidneys due to consumption of beer, wine, and other alcoholic beverages.)*

STOOL EXAMINATION: *(Indicated: Many Starch granules.)*
Gram Positive 20% *(normal - 35%)*   Gram Negative 80% *(normal - 65%)*
Bacillus Acidophilus - None Present.   B. Coli - Many.

152

alone can, at any time and in any way, become a cure-all. Far from it. If you have not given much thought to what you put into your body, you had better wake up and do some serious thinking. I would suggest that you study my book *Guide To Diet & Salad*. This book contains samples of my own meals, about which thousands of people of all ages have written to say have changed their lives for the better.

There is also another extremely important phase to be considered: the mental and spiritual side of our daily lives. Watch your mind carefully, study its vagaries, learn to control your thoughts. Whatever you do, don't go overboard on any philosophies which are not meant for intelligent Western people. The evanescent promises they make, and I must refer particularly to the cults of the East, all too often cause the victims to lose their sense of reality which we must have if we are to live in this world with a balanced mind. I am not speaking at random, but from a great many years of study and research of virtually every cult and religion prevalent in this day. I realize that this advice is useless to those who have been indoctrinated with elusive and fantastic expectations of achieving states of consciousness for which our body and mind are not intended. It is a mentally dangerous game which ensnares those who are not capable of thinking for themselves.

A lifetime of research has pointed out to me that Almighty God created each one of us for a purpose; it is up to us to discover that purpose.

As we cannot get the answers from thin air, we have been given the Bible, the infallible Word of God, as our guide. **Study it.**

Chapter 9.
The Filtering And Elimination Center

The Kidneys

We have two **kidneys**: one on the right, the middle of which is just about on the level of the 12th, or lowest rib, and one on the left, the center of which is just about on the level with the pyloric valve of the stomach. They are both located far back in the diaphragm region of the anatomy. They are only about 4½ inches long, about 2 inches wide, and about 1¼ inches thick. You can see what they look like by turning to the chapter on the adrenal glands in which the left kidney is illustrated.

The structure of the kidneys is very complex and this is not the place to go into the details. They are organs of elimination of liquid excreta, and the work they do is nothing short of amazing.

Every cell in the body, without exception, uses food to remain alive and to work for us. Each cell has its own process of assimilation and in the course of this process it has waste to eliminate. This waste is the endproduct of the process of metabolism. Metabolism is the process concerned with the building-up of the tissues and cells, as well as their destruction. Metabolism involves chemical changes in the tissues and their living cells, by which energy is produced for their vital functions. New material is assimilated to repair the worn-out cells. Thus, two steps are involved in metabolism. The constructive step is the building-up of nutritive substances into the more complex, living protoplasm. The destructive step causes the decomposition and oxidization of the constituents of protoplasm into simpler bodies, with the liberation of energy. While these processes of construction and destruction proceed together, one may predominate and obscure the other, causing an imbalance. It is obvious, when considering these processes of metabolism, that to deprive the tissues of living organic food results in the predominance of the destructive phase. When this proceeds beyond the limit of tolerance we have the seeds of toxemia springing up.

As the cells and tissues of the body use food and oxygen they naturally produce metabolic waste such as carbon dioxide. This, together with small amounts of water, is eliminated through the lungs. Carbon dioxide, as well as water and the secretion of some of the glands, is discarded through the eliminative system. The organs of the urinary system take care of the elimination of liquids which are segregated from metabolic substances.

The kidneys perform the complex task of extracting toxic waste of protein metabolism from the blood in the form of uric acid and urea. In addition, they extract from the blood and the lymph stream the cast-off and used-up minerals and other elements, as well as waste water.

Besides being active in these functions, the kidneys also regulate the activities which go on in their environment, such as quality and volume of water in

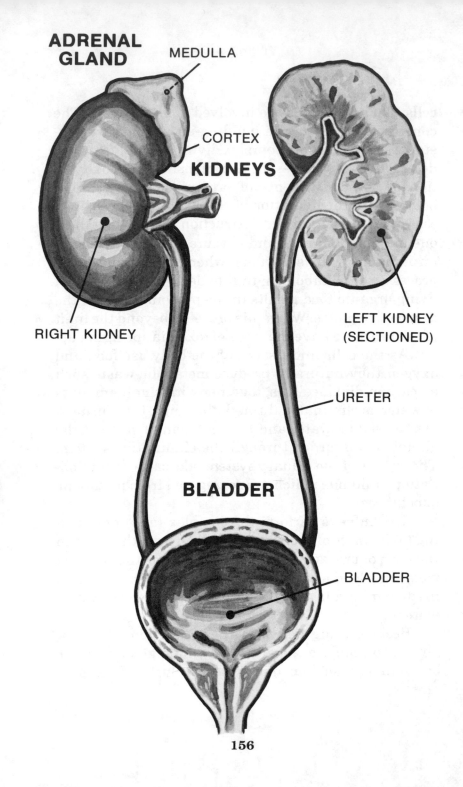

ADRENAL
GLAND

MEDULLA

CORTEX

KIDNEYS

RIGHT KIDNEY

LEFT KIDNEY
(SECTIONED)

URETER

BLADDER

BLADDER

156

the tissues, the osmosis process, and regulation of acid-balance.

The kidneys produce a secretion called rennin, which is taken up by the blood to be transmitted and used by the system when there is a need to constrict blood vessels.

Some secretions of the kidneys are involved in metabolic processes. The failure of the kidneys to secrete these, either wholly or in deficient quantities, results in deposits of uric acid. The resulting condition of uremia is caused by the retention of excreta in the blood which the kidneys should have eliminated. This is characterized by headaches, vertigo, vomiting, partial or total blindness, convulsions, coma, partial paralysis and a urinous odor of the breath.

Kidney stones are the result of the coagulation of mineral and other elements which form, in part, because of the composition of incompatible foods and foods cooked in oil or grease. The metabolism of the digestive system was not able to process these, and they were consequently excreted into the blood and passed on to the kidneys. When the blood carries such waste to the kidneys, they are not able to filter it for elimination in the urine, and stones are the result. We have seen kidney, as well as gall bladder, stones dissolved in a matter of two to four days by immersing them in a test tube filled with Cleaver's Tea, an herb readily obtained at health food stores. Herbalists frequently recommend Cleaver's Tea when there is any indication of kidney or gall bladder trouble.

Your kidneys are extremely valuable organs which

need watching because they respond to the condition of the colon. Alcohol, even the minute volumes in wines and beer, can play havoc with the kidneys. A very dear friend, who used to travel extensively in Europe, became accustomed to drinking wine with his meals. He died of uremic poisoning at the very early age of 56. The British, the Germans, as well as the Americans — nations which are the greatest consumers of beer — have the most serious and prolific kidney afflictions of any people in the world, although Italians, French and Latin people come a close second.

Because of the very nature of the excretions which pass through the kidneys, they are particularly susceptible to infections. It will be well worth your while to study carefully the chapter in this book entitled **Connective Tissue And Vitamin C**. The life it saves may be **your own!**

Prevention is a far better principle to live by than to try to obtain a cure. Colon irrigations are the best first step. Wash out the colon, then go on from there.

The Urinary Bladder

The **bladder** is a slightly distensible, membranous sac located in the pelvis in front of the rectum. It receives from the two ureters, the urine from the kidneys, discharging it from time to time into the urethra through an orifice closed by a sphincter, or muscular, valve.

Urine is the liquid excreta thrown off by the body. In a healthy condition, it is a clear, transparent fluid of an amber color and has a peculiar odor. Its average density is 1.02. The average amount excreted in 24 hours is from 35 to 50 ounces.

Chemically, urine is an aqueous solution of urea, creatine and uric acid, together with some hippuric acid, calcium, chloride, magnesium, phosphate, potassium, sodium and sulphate ions, as well as some peculiar pigments. It also should have an acid reaction. Normally it contains about 96% water and 4% solid matter. The average daily excretion of urine is about 30 grams of urea, 1 to 2 grams of creatine, 0.75 grams of uric acid and 16½ grams of salt. Abnormal urine may contain sugar as in diabetes, albumin as in Bright's disease, bile pigments as in jaundice, and blood in injuries or diseases of the kidneys or urinary passages. In the many urinalyses we have had done, the individuals habit of meat consumption was clearly indicated by an abnormal quantity of uric acid. It is obvious that the urinary bladder deserves a great deal of respect, as it is our reservoir of liquid excreta which, upon analysis, is likely to indicate the individual's eating, drinking and other habits. When having a urinalysis made, one should be sure of the honesty and integrity of the analyst.

The proximity of the urinary bladder to the descending and transverse colons, and particularly to the sigmoid flexure and the rectum, renders it particularly susceptible to any abnormality in any part of the colon. This is a very important matter to bear in mind throughout life. Yearly series of colon irrigations have been of inestimable value to uncountable numbers of our students in the past. One lovely couple — he is now in his 80's — called on me this very week. They were students in classes I gave more than 35 years ago. Their children had been brought up on the **Walker Program**, and they are proud of their son who, so far, is the only one in the state of California to be given a certificate of special merit for **never** having missed a single day at school — from the first day he was registered as a child, right through senior high and college. Does this not cause you to ponder on the lack of foresight in so many families who fail to teach their children the value of proper nutrition and of keeping the inside of their bodies cleansed? There is no substitute for health. Sickness and disease all too frequently have their beginnings in the colon; keep it clean —live healthy and longer.

An analysis of the excreta from the urinary bladder can readily indicate the condition of the colon and of the body as a whole. We always keep one or two rolls of Nitrazine Paper tape which is readily available at nearly every drug store. Using about one inch of this tape and letting some urine wet it, will indicate the acidity from 5 pH to 6, which is normally good, but when the color of it indicates from 6.5 pH or higher, it indicates alkalinity. However, never judge by a single excretion, as the acid-alkaline reading is likely to change within an hour or two.

If you want an analysis of your condition go to a qualified health practitioner, a chiropractor, a naturopathic physician or a therapist in good standing. The ancient Romans had a motto: "Verbum sat sapientis," which in our language means: "A word to the wise is sufficient."

Chapter 10.
Connective Tissue And Vitamin C

Colon irrigations are not by any means a "cure-all." Do not for one minute think they are.

The waste matter naturally collected in the colon and allowed to remain there longer than necessary is by nature subject to fermentation and putrefaction. It is this end-product of neglecting to keep the colon clean that produces a fertile ground for the propagation of pathogenic bacteria which are the precursors of sickness and disease.

As indicated on the *Colon Therapy Chart*, various parts of the anatomy are responsive to trouble caused by the accumulation of waste matter in that part of the colon which is related to its particular part of the anatomy. There are, however, some structural factors which may contribute to one or many disturbances which are entirely unrelated to the colon. Consider, for instance, the connective tissue system of the body. Connective tissues are the bond or cementing which anchors one body cell to another, making a web or a frame present in every particle of the body — the blood vessel walls, the nerve sheathing, the walls of the lymphatics, etc. Connective tissue also holds the various organs and glands of the body in their proper place. If the connective tissue of the kidneys break down, we have a floating kidney. When the connective tissue of the womb breaks down, we have a prolapsed womb. So it is throughout the whole body system. The connective tissues are of such vital importance to the body that when there is a weakening or a break down, trouble follows. A weakness of the wall tissues of the blood vessels manifests itself in an aneurysm. It may also develop an ulcer, and so on, almost ad infinitum.

The cleansing of the colon cannot remedy such disturbances of the connective tissues because they are absolutely dependent on a constant supply of **ascorbic acid**. Ascorbic acid is one of the substances which the body does not produce or manufacture within the system; it must be obtained by the body from the food with which it is nourished. Ascorbic acid is composed of molecules made up of 6 atoms of carbon, 8 atoms of hydrogen and 6 atoms of oxygen, which results in the formula, $C_6H_8O_6$. Ascorbic acid is known as Vitamin C and is present in varying amounts in many fruits and vegetables. The richest source of ascorbic acid comes from rose hips, from tree-ripened grapefruit, lemons and oranges, from Acerola cherries, guavas, bell peppers, pimiento peppers, brussel sprouts, mustard greens, dandelions and turnip greens. However, most fresh vegetables and fruits have varying amounts of Vitamin C.

A deficiency of ascorbic acid can have many adverse effects, such as failure of wounds to heal and weakening of bones, causing them to break easily and fail to mend in a reasonable time.

Ascorbic acid is the means by which hydrogen is

supplied to the digestive processes to burn the food we eat. This causes the necessary supply of carbon to be produced which the body needs to build the amino acids and other substances for which carbon is needed, including the maintenance of ascorbic acid when it is available in the system.

There are many ailments which afflict human beings which are either directly or indirectly due to a deficiency of ascorbic acid, or for which such deficiency is a contributing factor.

Taking everything into consideration, it is obvious that colon irrigations alone are not the complete answer to one's problems. It seems essential that ascorbic acid has an equally important role. A constant, daily, fresh supply of ascorbic acid is needed. In order to be sure to obtain this, we must consider our fresh vegetables and fruits — and their juices — an absolute **must** if we expect to regain and to maintain maximum health and to promote longevity with the avoidance of senility.

I will grant that there are times and circumstances when some ascorbic acid is needed in a hurry or an emergency. In such cases science comes to our aid, enabling us to obtain supplementary supplies of ascorbic acid. Under such circumstances it would naturally be foolhardy not to take advantage of such a commodity. It is good to bear in mind that synthetic products are never equal to the natural, nor are they ever as efficient or effective.

Ascorbic acid is one substance which the body cannot do without. There is no danger of taking too much ascorbic acid daily, so long as we take it in amounts spread throughout the day. When the daily amount is reached which the body needs and tolerates, Nature advises us that there is an excess by causing a mild case of diarrhea. It is then time to gradually reduce the dose, causing the diarrhea to cease.

When we understand that the body does not produce its own ascorbic acid to prevent damage and avoid afflictions of the body, we will realize that it would be very foolish to undertake prolonged fasts, extending beyond six or seven days. Prolonged fasts will deprive the body of foods which furnish ascorbic acid. Such deprivation can only result in degeneration of connective tissue, thus affecting nerves and muscles. Afflictions arising from this deprivation of such food may not materialize within months, or even within years, but it usually has long-range effects, such as conditions of premature senility, osteoporosis, Parkinson's Disease and a score of others.

Chapter 11.
The Ghastly Result Of Neglecting The Colon

Your body is your own responsibility!

Do you know that **today** there are more than one million people in the United States who, having failed to use colon irrigations, have had their colon unnecessarily amputated or sections of it removed? As long as they live, they will never have any control whatever over their bowel elimination!

Would **you** like to be in that predicament? Would you like to have your evacuation take place in a bag hanging, day and night, on your waist? If by accident or carelessness the bottom of the bag should open up or leak, the ghastly result is an embarrassing, filthy mess all down your leg, your foot and on the floor! It **can** happen! It **has** happened!

Let me ask you: **Why** do you continue to allow the 20, 30 or more years of corrupt feces and waste matter accumulated in layers on the inside of the wall of your colon to remain there, when it can be gradually removed with advantage and benefit to your health in general? No sewage system **of any kind** is immune from trouble if material is put into it which will eventually clog it up somewhere along the line. If the colon is neglected, each passing year has its ravaging effect on

THE ABNORMAL COLON

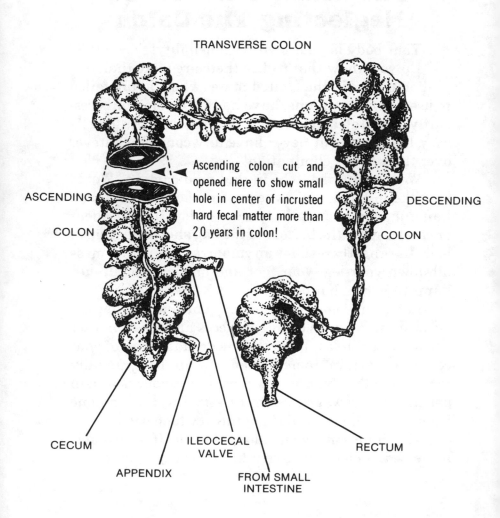

TRANSVERSE COLON

Ascending colon cut and opened here to show small hole in center of incrusted hard fecal matter more than 20 years in colon!

ASCENDING

COLON

DESCENDING

COLON

CECUM

ILEOCECAL VALVE

APPENDIX

FROM SMALL INTESTINE

RECTUM

the sewage system of the body. Watch your colon!

The accumulative putrefaction and fermentation which takes place in the colon causes offensive odors to escape from the body through the pores of the skin. You may not notice it— and few people do notice it on themselves — but others can detect this offensive emanation.

If your colon is still part of your midriff, thank God for it. Praise the Lord! If I were you, I would waste no time and go get a colon irrigation.

As I have already stated, more than one million people in our country have failed to cleanse their colon with irrigations. They have developed stomach and colon trouble and were rushed to the hospital "for an exploratory operation." When they came out from under the anaesthetic they discovered, to their ever-lasting regret and consternation, that a section of their colon had been removed, depriving them of any future control or normal function of their bowels.This is called a **colostomy**. Henceforth, the waste matter and feces would flow into, and be collected in, a bag which they would have to wear attached to their waist as long as they occupied their physical body.

Such people cannot afford to gamble on waiting until the bag is full before emptying it because they have no control over their evacuation. An accidental overflow would be too embarrassing to describe, and it would certainly never be forgotten —either by the victim or the bystander. This bag must be emptied, washed or replaced when little more than half-filled — as long as they live. Ghastly!

What a haunting, frightful, hideous prospect for any self-respecting constipated individual to contemplate! Wherever he or she is, wherever he or she goes, that bag **must** constantly be there, attached to the waist, emptied when necessary, every day and night, year after year, until the mortician removes it — permanently!

Is a Colostomy necessary? **No**, it is **not** necessary provided preventive steps are taken in time. What are these preventive measures? Don't just wait until your colon is completely blocked. Even when it is blocked it can be **washed out** by taking a series of colon irrigations.

We had a dear friend, an old lady, who was having trouble with her bowel movements. She went to the hospital for an examination. While she was under the anaesthetic the surgeon amputated her colon and performed a colostomy — without her knowledge and consent. Upon returning home she was aghast at what had been done to her. She prayed and beseeched Almighty God to take her out of this earthly life, which He did after she suffered many weeks of mental anguish.

Remember that a surgeon is trained to cut and amputate. It is not within his field to wash out the colon, or have it done. It is not surprising that nearly all those who have been afflicted with a colostomy never knew what was in store for them until they awakened from the operation; then, to their chagrin, they knew what a colostomy was.

Have you **any** idea of what a colostomy involves?

The following, in substance, is taken from instructions contained in the Colostomy Manual. I quote:

"You will be coping with appliances from now on (*for the rest of your life*).

The dismay over needing to carry this bag for the rest of your life is something every 'Colostomate' must overcome. (*If we thought* **dismay** *was not a normal reaction, we'd be kidding ourselves.*)

Discharge of the feces flows day and night (*without your being able to control it*) since there is no place except 'the bag' for it to go into.

There are no voluntary muscles involved, so you cannot control it.

Question: 'How can I get along without that control?' Answer: 'Thousands do!'

Healing of the hole in the side, made by the surgeon, progresses for several weeks after the operation.

'Disposable bags' means you can use a new one every day... but some go a day and a half and even longer between changes.

Anyone with sewing ability can alter a man's or a woman's garment to conceal the presence of the bag.

You may want to forego certain foods in order to: prevent blockage, to prevent a watery or inconvenient heavy discharge of fecal matter, to avoid excessive odor or gas.

Without the colon, dehydration and too

great a loss of sodium is likely. Call your doctor in case diarrhea bothers you.

Thirst will afflict you. Liquids are Nature's way to compensate for the loss of the water-absorbing colon.

Twin concerns are **odors** and **gas**! Occasional odor is 'normal'."

Study the foregoing. I have taken this from the Colostomy Manual which is published by the manufacturers of "the bag."

What is the expense involved in a colostomy? More than one million **victims** (Colostomates) spent more than **two billion dollars** for surgery and convalescence; but that is just the beginning.

The special bags cost presently from $12 to $15 for 30 bags. If you were to use one bag a day (which many **must**) the cost would be from about $150 to $200 a year, as long as you live. You won't be able to go **anywhere** unless you have a supply of bags to take with you. The likelihood of not being able to get bags would create a nightmare.

Don't risk a colostomy. It is not worth it. Keep your high enema outfit handy, and don't hesitate to use it (see my book *Become Younger*). Don't let distances prevent having colon irrigations when necessary. It's your own body, and you are responsible for it.

Let this ghastly spectre of a colostomy, having a bag half-filled with filthy feces hang at your waist day and night, remind you that any advice or recommendation to avoid a colon irrigation is utterly false, misleading and absolutely devoid of basis in fact or in common sense. I shall maintain to my dying day that any person who opposes, censures or raves against cleansing the colon by this means, is afflicted with what the ancient Romans classified as "Non Compos Mentis." Obviously such people do not differentiate between the clean and the filthy. It is through such lack of perception that more than one million people today defecate without any voluntary control whatever into that filthy bag which they have to empty by hand and clean out or replace, every single day as long as they live.

Be prudent. Be wise. Prevention is better than **no cure**. Don't take **my** word for it. Prove it yourself by taking a number of colonics. My own life will not be affected in the least by what you do or don't do. BUT the life it may save may be **your own**.

My People Perish
For Lack Of Knowledge

Hosea 4:6

Tell me not in doleful tones
    My text is for the birds and drones.
That your colon and its illness
    Is your own, and not my business.

Read this book, my Reader Friend,
    Read it to the very end.
Study every illustration.
    Don't give rein to imagination.

You may find I'm not so wrong
    And you'll change to a different song.
That at least is what I hope for.
    There's no cure the which to dope for.

Get your colon irrigation;
    Get that wonderful sensation
Feeling clean inside and out.
    This should banish every doubt.

Sing your Hallelujah song,
    Know that now it won't be long
When aches and pains that left you aghast
    Are nightmares of the recent past.

N. W. Walker

*INDEX

*Note: Main entries in alphabetical order.
Sub-entries in page sequence.*

176

177

Thyroid —
location of, 89
size of, 89
in menstruation, 89
function of, 89
iodine requirement, 89, 90, 91
relationship to tonsils, 91
controlled by pituitary glands, 93

Thyroxin —
iodine in, 91
results of iodine insufficiency, 91
metabolism dependent on, 93

Tissues —
also see Cells
connective, 161

Tonsils —
area in colon involved with, 61, 64
definition of, 61
minimized importance of, 61
appendix related to, 63, 64
relationship to colon cleanliness, 63, 69
danger in removal, 64, 143
example of removal, 64
relationship to reproductive organs, 64, 67
loss of sexual dynamism, 66, 67
British youth vs. Italian youth, 66
results of tonsillectomies, 68, 143, 144
inflammed, indication of toxicity, 144

Tonsillectomy —
examples of, 64, 65, 66, 70
statistics on, 69

Toxemia —
outcome of failure to expel feces, 5
definition of, 13

Toxic —
cells & tissues, 8

Toxicity —
coating of slime generates, 14

Trace Elements —
present in spinal fluid, 78
alfalfa, richest source, 79

Trachea —
location of, 81
size of, 81
affected by mucus, 81

Transverse Colon —
location of, 35
function of, 35

Tuberculosis, 82

Tympanum, 53

Ulcers, 162

Universities —
Vienna, 63
Berlin, 63

Uremia, 157

Urethra —
definition of, 141
inflammation of, 141

Uric Acid —
result of meat consumption, 159

Uric Acid Crystals —
accumulation of, 18
indication of fecal accumulation, 18

Urine —
description of, 158, 159
abnormal, 159
analysis shows, 159, 160

Uterus —
purpose of, 143
description of, 144, 146
location of, 144
prolapse of, 144
cancer of, 145

Vagina —
location of, 146

Vagus Nerve —
controls cardiac sphincter, 110

Vegetable —
raw, value of, 118

Vegetable Juices —
see Juices

Veins —
varicose, 47

Ventricle, Third, 43

Veteran, 23

Veteran's Hospital, 23

Vibrations —
in electric wires, 31
cosmic, in male body, 31
cosmic, in female body, 31
in color, 32
in hemoglobin, 32
in lungs, 32
in pituitary glands, 32
in ears, 32
in sickness, 32
in health, 32
as a diagnostic tool, 32, 33

Villi, 115, 116

Vitamin —
A, B1, B2, B6, C, D, E, K, 117
K, 117, 119

Vitamin C —
depletion with colds, 57
relationship to connective tissue, 49
composition of, 117, 162
connective tissues dependent upon, 162
sources of, 162
results of deficiencies in, 162
function within body, 163
synthetic form, 163
symptoms of excess, 164

Vitamins —
atoms in, 117, 118
related to liver, 117
volume of, in grams, 118

Walker Program, 131, 132, 138, 160

Walking —
diaphragm exercise, 106

Washington —
deficiency of iodine in, 92
colon irrigations for iodine deficiency, 92

Water —
natural elements, 19
composition of, 19
body, distilled, 40, 93
function of, in body, 40
damage to optic system, 47
lime in, 47
balance, in body, 93
results of insufficient, in body, 93
distilled, 132

Water Can Undermine Your Health, 48

West Virginia —
Clendenin, 89

Windpipe, 86

Wine —
see Alcohol

Wisconsin —
deficiency of iodine in, 92
colon irrigations for iodine deficiency, 92

Womb —
prolapsed, 162

Worms —
shown in X-ray, 39, 131, 151
in cecum pouch, 39, 131
example of, 40

Wounds —
failure to heal, 162

X ray —
of colon, for irrigation, 20
as indication of colon condition, 22, 23, 51
of colon, shows "V" form, 39
of colon, showing disturbance of
mammary glands, 150

179

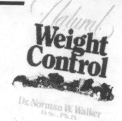
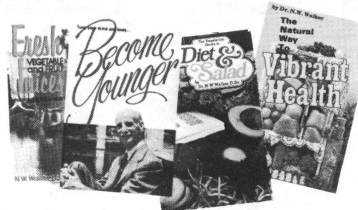

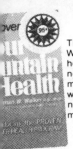

Discover Your
Fountain of Health

This new book is a capsule version of Dr. Walker's complete program for better health. It will give you new knowledge -- and new hope -- with easy-to-follow guides for maintaining or renewing your health. You will discover how to live with a vitality you've never experienced before. You ARE the master of your fate.

.95¢

Colon Health:
the Key to a Vibrant Life

This book shows how every organ, gland and cell in the body is affected by the condition of the large intestine -- the colon, which is the body's "sewage system." When it becomes clogged with waste and corruption, problems develop. The book explains the importance of colon care and how to accomplish colon hygiene for a longer, healthier life.

$4.95

Water Can Undermine
Your Health

ater pollution is a major problem in tually every community in the country. is book gives the shocking facts on how e water we drink can affect our health. It scusses the impurities in drinking water at can cause varicose veins, arthritis, ncer and even heart attacks. How to avoid e problems that polluted water can create.

$4.95

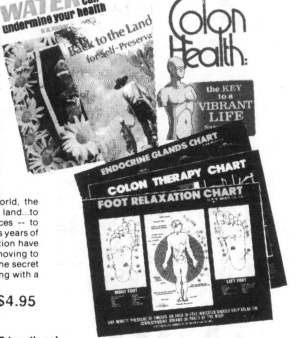

Back to the Land
for Self-Preservation

In today's hectic and complex world, the time has come to get back to the land...to learn by other people's experiences -- to profit by their mistakes. Dr. Walker's years of working for better health and nutrition have led him to explore the wisdom of moving to the COUNTRY, there to discover the secret of peace and regeneration and living with a purpose!

$4.95

Dr. Walker's Educational
Wall Charts
17" x 22" in color

FOOT RELAXATION - The Soles of your Feet can help relax tension in various parts of your body. This chart shows the Zones on the Soles of the Feet in relation to the rest of the body.

ENDOCRINE GLANDS - See where they are located in your body - their innumerable functions, what elements compose them, what Juices nourish them.

blished by

SULLIVAN
OODSIDE
COMPANY

COLON THERAPY - This is the most complete chart of the human Colon. It indicates the relation of nerve endings from head to foot registered in the Colon, and should alert you to study your own condition and to do something about it.

$5.00 each

PLEASE SHIP AT ONCE:

	copies	each	extension
NATURAL WEIGHT CONTROL	_____	@ 4.95	$ _____
COLON HEALTH — Vibrant Life	_____	@ 4.95	_____
VIBRANT HEALTH-Possible Dream	_____	@ 4.95	_____
FRESH VEGETABLE AND FRUIT JUICES	_____	@ 4.95	_____
BECOME YOUNGER	_____	@ 4.95	_____
DIET & SALAD SUGGESTIONS, Revised	_____	@ 4.95	_____
WATER CAN UNDERMINE YOUR HEALTH	_____	@ 4.95	_____
BACK TO THE LAND	_____	@ 4.95	_____
CHARTS:			
Endocrine Glands	_____	@ 5.00	_____
Colon Therapy	_____	@ 5.00	_____
Foot Relaxation	_____	@ 5.00	_____

Please add $1.00 per copy for postage & handling _____

ENCLOSED IS MY ☐ CHECK ☐ CASH FOR ...... $ _____

Please Remit in U.S. Dollars

NAME _____

STREET ADDRESS _____

CITY _____

STATE _____ ZIP _____

You
Save Postage
when buying from
Health Food &
Book Stores!

or order from:

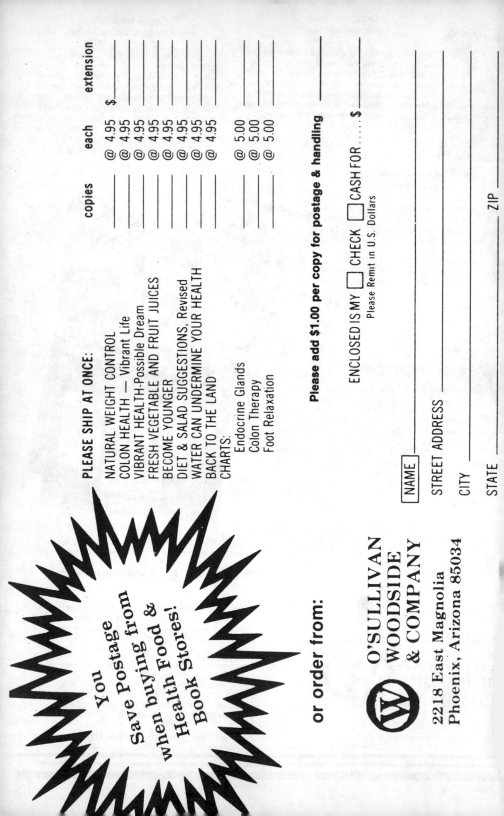

**O'SULLIVAN
WOODSIDE
& COMPANY**

2218 East Magnolia
Phoenix, Arizona 85034